EAT LIKE A

Trophy Model

ANGELA BOWIE

Order this book online at www.trafford.com
or email orders@trafford.com

Most Trafford titles are also available at major online book retailers.

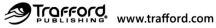 www.trafford.com

North America & international
toll-free: 1 888 232 4444 (USA & Canada)
fax: 812 355 4082

Our mission is to efficiently provide the world's finest, most comprehensive book publishing service, enabling every author to experience success. To find out how to publish your book, your way, and have it available worldwide, visit us online at www.trafford.com

Scripture quotations marked KJV are from the Holy Bible, King James Version (Authorized Version). First published in 1611. Quoted from the KJV Classic Reference Bible, Copyright © 1983 by The Zondervan Corporation.

Scripture quotations marked NIV are taken from the Holy Bible, New International Version®. NIV®. Copyright © 1973, 1978, 1984 by International Bible Society. Used by permission of Zondervan. All rights reserved.

ISBN: 978-1-4907-9727-4 (sc)
         978-1-4907-9726-7 (e)

Print information available on the last page.

Trafford rev. 09/26/2019

Contents

$\mathcal{I}$ntroduction

Are you a model or are you considering a career as one?

Is modeling not for you but you would like to have the body of one?

Have you considered that the food you eat is a vital part of the process?

Losing weight or keeping trim is a goal that many women have, whether they want to become a famous model or not. The benefits to be gained are enormous, from the positive effects on our health, complexion, energy and body shape, so it's well worth it. The good news is that almost anyone can do it.

Inside this book, **Eat Like a Trophy Model,** you will discover a range of delicious low carb, seafood recipes that don't skimp on flavor but provide you with a balanced diet that promotes weight loss, including dishes like:

> **Cajun scallops**
> **Tuna salad**
> **Shrimp egg rolls**
> **Superwoman Salmon**
> **Cioppino**
> **Cajun lobster tails**
> **Pan-fried sea bass with tomato and basil**
> **And many more...**

Written by a successful model with 25 years of experience in making sure she ate the right things, **Eat Like a Trophy Model** aims to motivate women of all ages to adopt a healthy eating routine and lifestyle.

Everything starts with the food you eat and by following the principles in this book you can look like a Trophy Model too.

Trophy Model Motto: Start you day with grapes and end it with wine

Cajun Scallops

Cooking time: 15 minutes

Servings: 2

Ingredients:

- ¾ lbs fresh scallops
- 1 teaspoon olive oil
- 1 red onion, sliced
- 1 teaspoon Cajun seasoning

- ½ teaspoon ground black pepper
- 1 teaspoon butter
- 1 garlic clove
- 2 teaspoons hot sauce

Instructions:

1. Preheat oil in a skillet over high heat. Add onion, Cajun seasoning and pepper and sauté for about 3 minutes.
2. Add butter and garlic; cook for 30 seconds more. Add scallops and cook for 2 minutes each side or until browned. Sprinkle with hot sauce, optional. Enjoy with your favorite side dish.

Nutritional info (per serving): 225 calories; 5.7 g fat; 12.5 g carbohydrate; 29.8 g protein

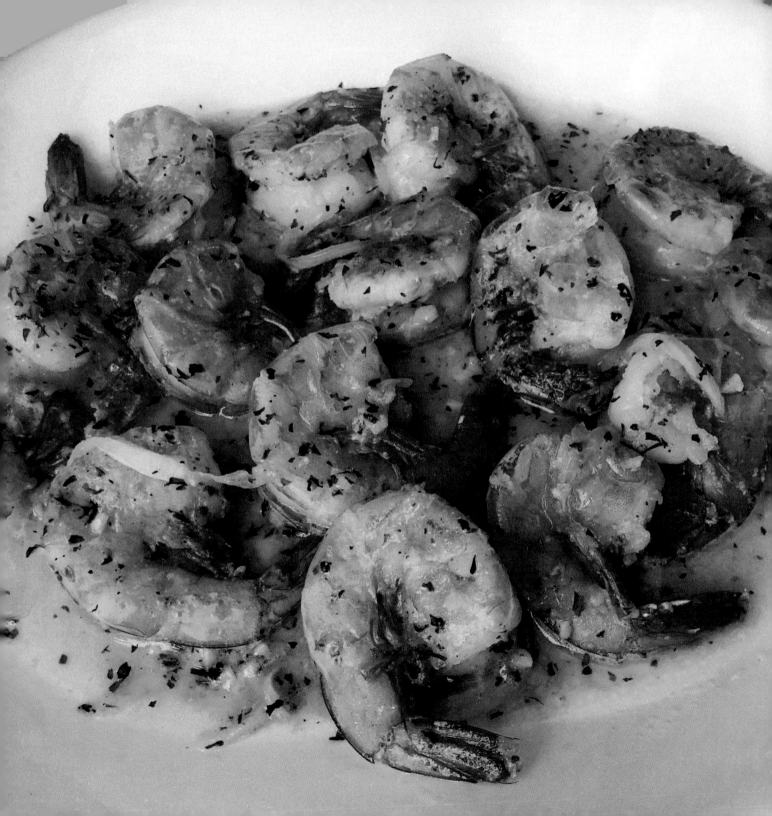

Butter Garlic Shrimp with Lemon Aioli

Cooking time: 20 minutes

Servings: 8

Ingredients:

For the Aioli:

- ½ cup mayonnaise
- 2 garlic cloves, chopped
- 1 tablespoon lemon juice
- 1 teaspoon lemon zest

For the Shrimp:

- 1 lb extra-large shrimp, uncooked, deveined, peeled, with tails left on
- 6 tablespoons butter
- 2 tablespoons Worcestershire sauce
- 1 teaspoon crushed red pepper flakes
- 3 garlic cloves, chopped
- 16 slices whole wheat bread
- 1 tablespoon Italian parsley leaves, chopped

Instructions:

1. Mix all Aioli ingredients in a bowl and beat well.
2. Preheat the broiler. Spray a baking pan with cooking spray.
3. Preheat butter in a saucepan over medium heat and melt it. Remove from heat, add Worcestershire sauce, pepper flakes and 3 garlic cloves. Brush each bread slice with the butter mixture from both sides, place on the baking pan and broil for 2 minutes per side. Transfer to a plate.
4. Add shrimp to the same pan, pour the remaining butter mixture on top and broil for 4-6 minutes. Serve topped with parsley, with sauce and bread on the side.

Nutritional info (per serving): 200 calories; 19 g fat; 13 g carbohydrate; 12 g protein

Fish Taco Bites

Cooking time: 20 minutes

Servings: 36

Ingredients:

- 1 lb cod filet
- ¼ cup all-purpose flour
- 8 oz cream cheese, softened
- ½ cup mayonnaise
- 2 tablespoons milk
- 2 tablespoons lemon juice

- ½ teaspoon garlic salt
- Salt, pepper, to taste
- 2 tablespoons olive oil
- 36 tortilla chip scoops
- ½ cup radishes, sliced
- ¼ cup cilantro, chopped

Instructions:

1. Beat mayonnaise, milk, lemon juice and garlic salt in a bowl until smooth. Cover and refrigerate for at least 30 minutes.

2. Season fish with salt and pepper on both sides. Dip the fillet into flour.

3. Preheat the olive oil in a large skillet over medium heat and add cod filet, cook for 3-5 minutes per side. Let cool and chop into bite sized pieces.

4. Place the tortilla chips on a plate. Top with cream cheese mixture, fish, radish and cilantro. Serve.

Nutritional info (per serving): 63 calories; 4 g fat; 4 g carbohydrate; 3 g protein

Crispy Coconut Shrimp

Cooking time: 30 minutes

Servings: 4

Ingredients:

- 1 lb shrimp, peeled, deveined
- 2 eggs
- 1 cup original Bisquick mix
- 1 cup shredded coconut

- ¼ teaspoon ground ginger
- ¼ teaspoon ground cardamom
- ¼ teaspoon salt
- 1 ½ cups coconut oil

For the Sauce:

- ⅓ cup orange marmalade
- ⅓ cup apricot preserves

- 1 tablespoon water
- ½ teaspoon soy sauce

Instructions:

1. Mix all sauce ingredients in a microwavable bowl and microwave on High for 30-50 seconds. Stir well to combine.
2. Beat eggs in a bowl. In a separate bowl, mix Bisquick mix, coconut, ginger, cardamom and salt.
3. Preheat oil in a skillet over medium heat. Dip each shrimp into eggs, then into Bisquick mixture and cook in the skillet for about 2 minutes per side. Transfer to a plate lined with paper towels.
4. Serve with the sauce.

Nutritional info (per serving): 199 calories; 16.2 g fat; 9.9 g carbohydrate; 5.3 g protein

Cajun Shrimp Scampi Rice

Cooking time: 40 minutes

Servings: 4

Ingredients:

For the Rice:

- 2 ½ cups chicken broth
- 1 cup long grain rice
- ½ cup onion, diced
- ¼ cup celery, diced
- ¼ cup bell pepper, diced
- 1 garlic clove, minced

- 3 tablespoons butter
- ¼ teaspoon paprika
- ¼ teaspoon cayenne pepper
- ½ teaspoon dried oregano
- ½ teaspoon dried basil
- Salt, pepper, to taste

For the Shrimp:

- 1 lb large shrimp, peeled and deveined
- 2 teaspoons Cajun seasoning
- 1 tablespoon olive oil
- 2 teaspoons garlic, minced

- 2 tablespoons butter
- ¼ cup white wine
- 1 tablespoon lemon juice
- Salt, pepper, to taste

Instructions:

1. Preheat butter in a pot over medium heat. Add onion, celery, bell pepper and garlic. Cook for about 5 minutes. Add paprika, cayenne pepper, oregano and basil and stir well.

2. Add rice and stir well to coat. Add chicken broth, cover the pot and simmer for about 15-20 minutes. Fluff rice with a fork once cooked.

3. Rub shrimp with Cajun seasoning, salt and pepper. Preheat oil in a pan over medium heat, add shrimp and cook for 2-3 minutes. Remove from pan and set aside.

4. Add garlic to the same pan, cook for 1 minute and add butter. Pour white wine, lemon zest and lemon juice to the pot. Cook until thickened. Toss the shrimp and parsley with the sauce. Serve over the rice.

Nutritional info (per serving): 329 calories; 12 g fat; 21 g carbohydrate; 44 g protein

Garlicky Tiger Prawns

Cooking time: 10 minutes

Servings: 4

Ingredients:

- 1 ½ lbs tiger prawns, shell-on
- 3 oz butter, melted
- 4 garlic cloves, peeled and crushed
- 1 tablespoon fresh parsley, chopped
- ½ lemon, zested and juiced
- 1 lemon, sliced, for serving
- Salt, pepper, to taste

Instructions:

1. Preheat the oven to 450 degrees F. Prepare a baking dish and coat with cooking spray.
2. Peel the prawns from one side and leave the tails on. Butterfly each prawn with a sharp knife.
3. Mix butter, garlic, lemon juice and zest in a bowl. Brush each prawn with the butter mixture and place into the baking dish. Bake for 6-7 minutes and serve topped with parsley.

Nutritional info (per serving): 158 calories; 8 g fat; 4 g carbohydrate; 12 g protein

Spinach Artichoke Dip

Cooking time: 25 minutes

Servings: 12

Ingredients:

- 8 oz cream cheese, softened
- 1 can (14 oz) artichoke hearts, drained, chopped
- ½ cup frozen spinach, drained
- ¼ cup mayo
- ¼ cup Parmesan, grated

- ¼ cup Mozzarella cheese, grated
- 1 garlic clove, minced
- ¼ cup Romano cheese, grated
- ½ teaspoon dried basil
- Salt, pepper, to taste

Instructions:

1. Preheat the oven to 350 F. Lightly grease a small baking dish.
2. Mix cream cheese, mayonnaise, Parmesan cheese, Romano cheese, garlic, basil, salt and pepper in a bowl. Gently stir in artichoke hearts and spinach.
3. Transfer the mixture to the prepared baking dish. Top with mozzarella cheese and bake for 25 minutes.

Nutritional info (per serving): 134 calories; 11.7 g fat; 3.4 g carbohydrate; 4.4 g protein

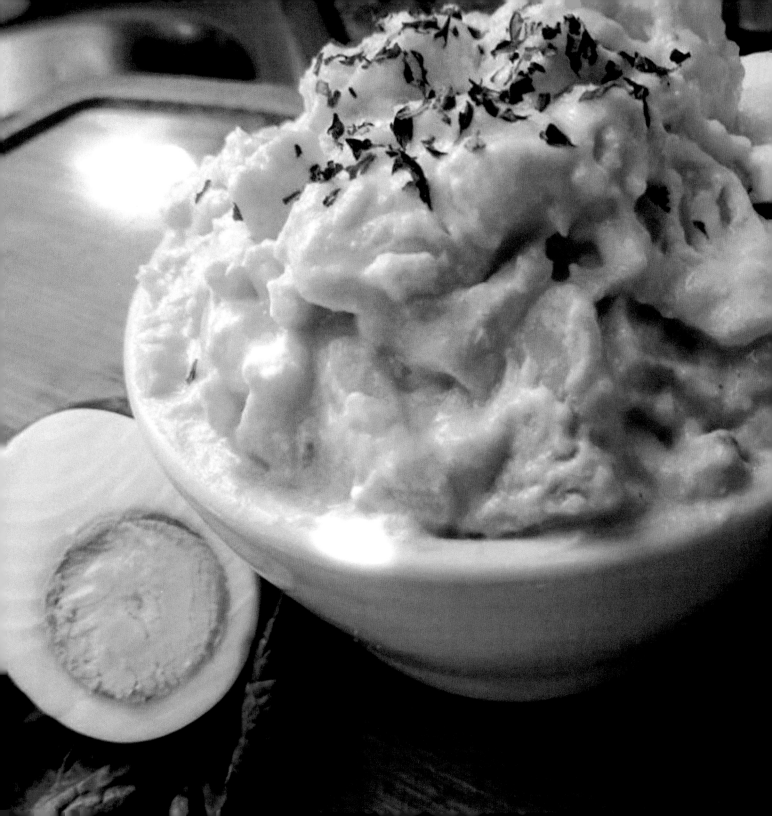

Evon's Heavenly Deviled Egg Potato Salad

Cooking time: 15 minutes

Servings: 2

Ingredients:

- 3 lbs Yukon gold potatoes, peeled and chopped
- 1 carrot
- ½ cup sweet relish
- 1 cup mayonnaise
- 3 tablespoons mustard

- 6 eggs, hard-boiled, peeled and chopped
- 3 celery ribs, sliced
- 6 scallions, sliced
- ⅓ cup parsley, chopped
- 1 jar (4 oz) diced pimentos, drained
- Salt, pepper, to taste

Instructions:

1. Add potatoes and carrot to a saucepan and cover with water, add salt. Bring to a boil and cook for about 4-5 minutes until tender. Drain and let cool, then chop.

2. Mix mayo, mustard, potatoes, eggs, celery, scallions, relish, parsley and pimentos. Stir well to combine everything, season with salt and pepper and serve.

Nutritional info (per serving): 333 calories; 16 g fat; 8 g carbohydrate; 18 g protein

Mini Pineapple Rum Shrimp Tostadas

Cooking time: 15 minutes

Servings: 8

Ingredients:

- 16 small shrimp, peeled and deveined
- 4 soft flour tortillas
- 1 cup pineapple, chopped
- ¼ cup brown sugar
- 1 tablespoon lime juice
- 1 teaspoon taco seasoning mix
- ½ teaspoon salt
- 2 tablespoons rum
- 1 avocado, diced
- 1 cup cabbage, shredded
- ¼ cup cilantro, chopped

Instructions:

1. Cut out 16 small circles from tortillas.
2. Mix brown sugar, lime juice, rum and seasoning in a bowl. Add shrimp and toss well to coat. Let rest for about 15 minutes.
3. Mix shredded cabbage with lime juice and olive oil in a separate bowl.
4. Thread the shrimps onto the skewers. Preheat the grill to medium high and grill the shrimp for 1-2 minutes per side. Place tortillas on the grill and cook for about 1 minute per side.
5. Place pineapple, red onion and avocado on a grill pan and cook until slightly browned.
6. Place cabbage on each tortilla and top with pineapple, avocado and red onion. Top with shrimp and cilantro.

Nutritional info (per serving): 212 calories; 7.2 g fat; 22.7 g carbohydrate; 12.7 g protein

Shrimp and Cucumber Rounds

Cooking time: 5 minutes

Servings: 36

Ingredients:

- ½ lb shrimp, cooked, peeled, deveined and chopped
- 1 English cucumber, thickly sliced
- ½ cup reduced-fat mayonnaise
- 2 green onions, sliced
- 1 celery rib, chopped
- 1 teaspoon dill pickle relish
- A pinch of cayenne pepper

Instructions:

1. Mix shrimp, mayo, green onions, celery, dill relish and cayenne pepper in a bowl. Cover and refrigerate for at least 30 minutes.
2. Spoon the mixture on top of cucumber slices and serve.

Nutritional info (per serving): 20 calories; 1 g fat; 1 g carbohydrate; 1 g protein

Tuna Salad

Cooking time: 5 minutes

Servings: 4

Ingredients:

- 2 cans tuna, drained
- ½ cup sweet relish
- 2 tablespoons mayonnaise
- 2 tablespoons plain Greek yogurt
- ½ lemon, juiced
- ½ teaspoon hot sauce
- ¼ red onion, chopped
- 2 dill pickles, chopped
- Lettuce, for serving
- Bread, for serving
- Salt, pepper, to taste
- 2 boiled eggs, chopped

Instructions:

1. Whisk mayonnaise, yogurt, lemon juice and hot sauce in a bowl.
2. Add tuna to the mayo mixture, stir well to combine.
3. Add sweet relish, eggs red onion and pickles, toss to combine. Season with salt and pepper. Serve on lettuce with bread.

Nutritional info (per serving): 281 calories; 11.2 g fat; 7.6 g carbohydrate; 35.4 g protein

Im sure some people don't like guacomole, but they probably don't have a friend named Hosea

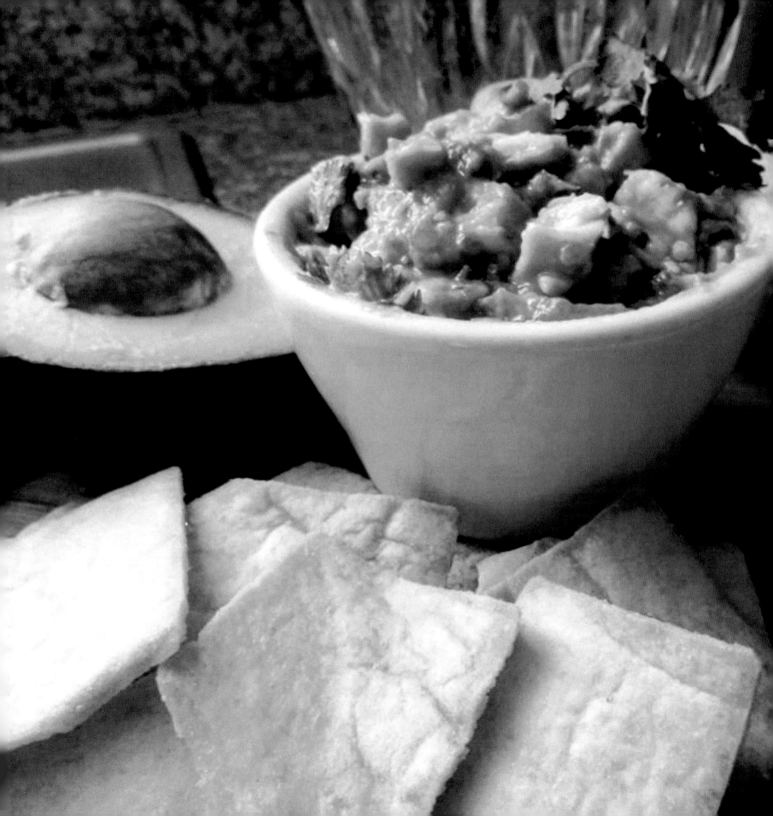

Rhea's Chunky Guacamole

Cooking time: 5 minutes

Servings: 4

Ingredients:

- 2 avocados
- ¼ cup red onion, minced
- 1 plum tomato, diced
- 1 teaspoon jalapeno, chopped
- ¼ cup cilantro, chopped
- ½ teaspoon salt

Instructions:

1. Chop one avocado and add the other one to a blender, process until smooth.
2. Mix pureed avocado with chopped avocado, add onion, tomato, jalapeno, cilantro and salt. Stir to combine and serve.

Nutritional info (per serving): 165 calories; 8 g fat; 11 g carbohydrate; 10 g protein

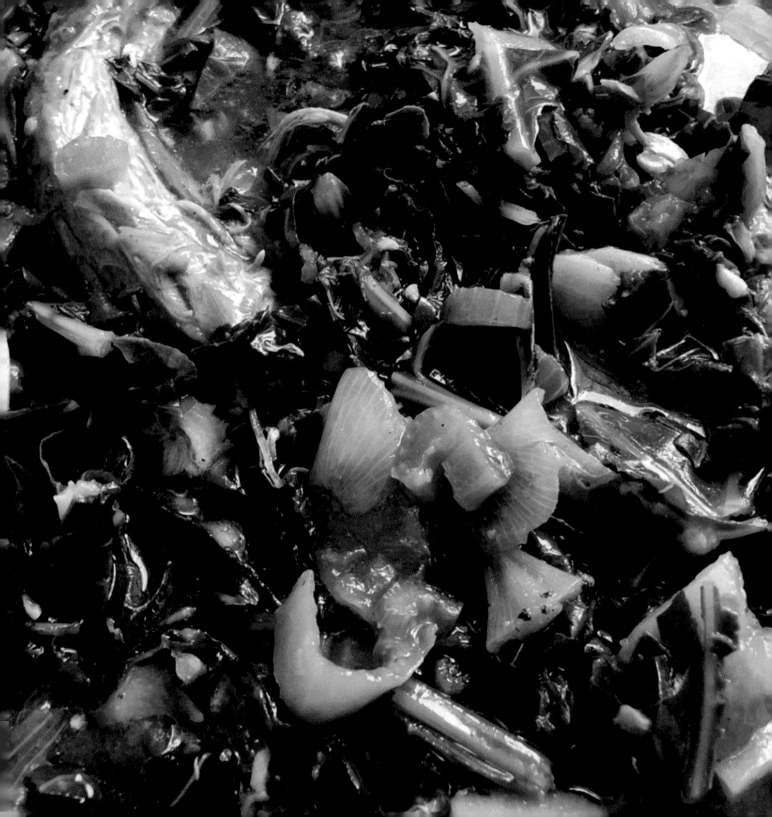

PawPaw's Southern Mixed Greens

Cooking time: 3 hours

Servings: 4

Ingredients:

- 2 bunches collard greens
- 2 bunches turnip greens & bottoms
- 2 bunches mustard greens
- 1 lb smoked turkey
- 1 teaspoon garlic, minced
- ½ onion, sliced

- 1 teaspoon paprika
- 1 teaspoon Creole seasoning
- A pinch red pepper flakes
- 2 cup chicken or vegetable broth
- 2 tablespoons apple cider vinegar
- Salt, pepper, to taste

Instructions:

1. Bring a pot of water with smoked turkey to a boil and cook over low heat for about 45 minutes.
2. Preheat the stock in a saucepan over medium heat. Add all the spices and all the greens, add garlic, onion and meat. Peel and slice the turnip bottoms and add with greens.
3. Cover the lid and cook on low heat for 2 ½ hours, stirring every 30 minutes. Serve.

Nutritional info (per serving): 234 calories; 21 g fat; 10 g carbohydrate; 25 g protein

Shrimp Salad with Green Curry Dressing

Cooking time: 15 minutes

Servings: 4

Ingredients:

- 1 lb large shrimp, cooked
- 8 oz mixed lettuces, chopped
- ¼ cup fresh lime juice
- ¼ cup canola oil
- 2 tablespoons green curry paste
- 1 cup cilantro leaves
- 1 cup mint leaves
- 1 cup carrot, sliced
- ½ cup red onion, sliced
- Salt, to taste
- Roasted peanuts, chopped, for serving

Instructions:

1. Whisk lime juice, oil and green curry paste in a bowl.
2. Add the shrimp, mixed lettuces, cilantro, mint, carrot and onion and toss well to combine. Season with salt and toss again.
3. Serve topped with chopped roasted peanuts and serve.

Nutritional info (per serving): 264 calories; 15.4 g fat; 10.8 g carbohydrate; 22.6 g protein

Smoked Salmon Salad

Cooking time: 15 minutes

Servings: 4

Ingredients:

- 8 cups baby spinach
- 6 oz smoked salmon, sliced
- 1 English cucumber, peeled, halved lengthwise, seeded and sliced
- 4 radishes, halved and sliced

- 3 tablespoons extra-virgin olive oil
- 2 tablespoons fresh lemon juice
- 2 tablespoon dill, chopped
- 2 scallions, sliced
- Salt, pepper, to taste

Instructions:

1. Whisk olive oil, lemon juice and dill in a bowl, season with salt and pepper.
2. Add spinach, smoked salmon, cucumber, radishes and scallions and toss well to combine. Serve.

Nutritional info (per serving): 174 calories; 12.8 g fat; 6.6 g carbohydrate; 10.5 g protein

Butter and Lemon Scallops

Cooking time: 10 minutes

Servings: 4

Ingredients:

- 1 lb scallops

For the Sauce:

- 2 tablespoons butter, unsalted
- 2 garlic cloves, minced
- 1 lemon, juiced

- 1 tablespoon butter, unsalted

- 2 tablespoons fresh parsley leaves, chopped
- Sea salt, pepper, to taste

Instructions:

1. Preheat butter in a skillet over medium heat. Season scallops with salt and pepper and add to the skillet.
2. Cook for about 1-2 minutes per side. Transfer to a plate.
3. Add the butter for the sauce to a skillet. Add garlic and cook for about 1 minute. Add lemon juice, parsley, salt and pepper.
4. Serve scallops with butter sauce.

Nutritional info (per serving): 183 calories; 9.9 g fat; 1.6 g carbohydrate; 21.3 g protein

If you are willing and obedient, you will eat the good things of the land- Isaiah 1:19

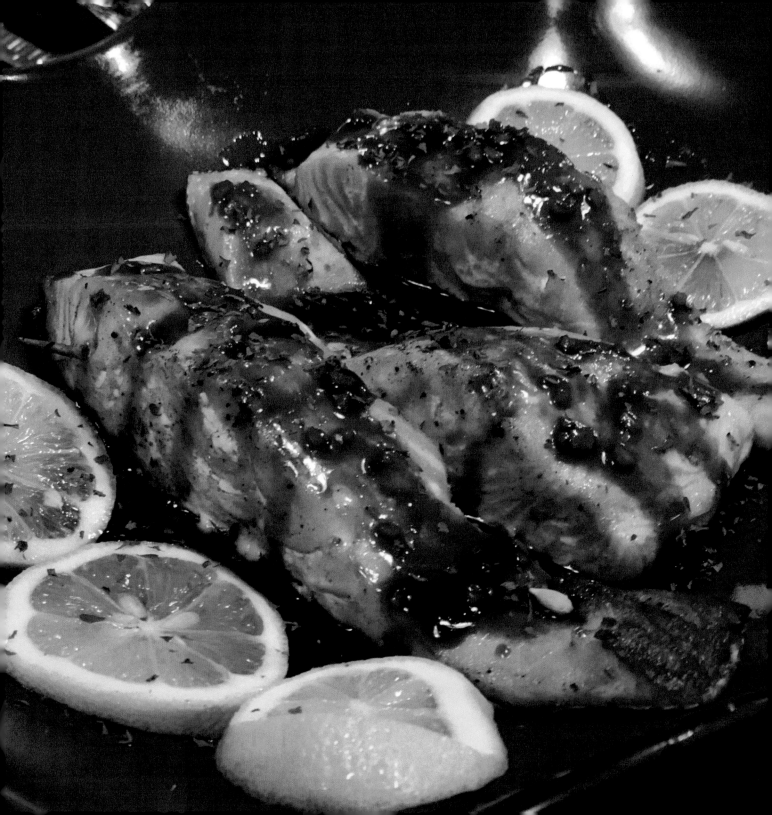

Tasha's Teriyaki salmon

Cooking time: 25 minutes

Servings: 4

Ingredients:

- 4 salmon fillets
- 3 tablespoons soy sauce
- 1 piece (1 inch) fresh ginger, sliced
- 2 garlic cloves, minced

- 2 tablespoons honey
- 1 tablespoon rice wine
- 2 tablespoons olive oil
- Sea salt, pepper, to taste

Instructions:

1. Mix ginger, garlic, soy sauce, honey, rice wine and oil in a bowl.
2. Season salmon with salt and pepper and coat with the soy sauce mixture. Refrigerate for at least 1 hour.
3. Preheat a splash of oil in a skillet over medium heat. Add salmon and cook for about 3-4 minutes per side. Serve salmon with the sauce on top.

Nutritional info (per serving): 147 calories; 11 g fat; 9 g carbohydrate; 25 g protein

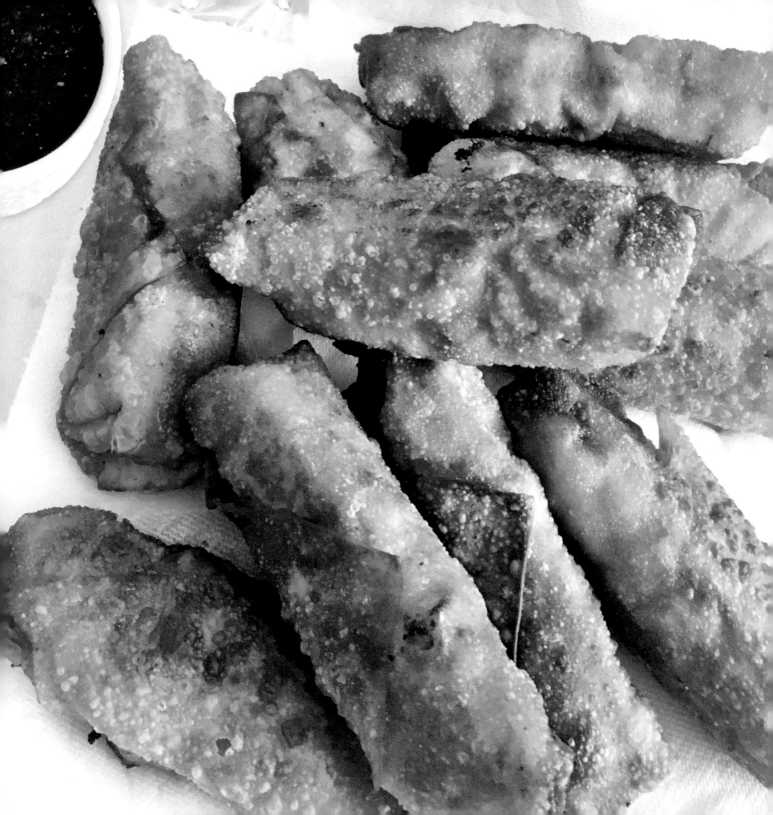

Shrimp Egg Rolls

Cooking time: 10 minutes

Servings: 18

Ingredients:

- 1 lb medium shrimp, peeled, deveined and chopped
- 18 egg roll wrappers
- 1 cup vegetable oil
- 3 cups coleslaw mix
- ½ cup bean sprouts
- 1 celery stalk, diced

- 2 green onions, sliced
- 2 garlic cloves, minced
- 1 tablespoon reduced sodium soy sauce
- 1 tablespoon oyster sauce
- 1 tablespoon ginger, grated
- 1 teaspoon sesame oil
- 1 teaspoon Sriracha

Instructions:

1. Mix shrimp, coleslaw mix, bean sprouts, celery, green onions, garlic, soy sauce, oyster sauce, ginger, sesame oil and Sriracha in a bowl.
2. Place shrimp mixture into the center of each egg wrapper and wrap. Rub the edges of the wrapper with water, pressing to seal.
3. Preheat vegetable oil in a skillet over medium high heat. Add egg rolls to the skillet and cook for about 2-3 minutes until golden brown. Serve.

Nutritional info (per serving): 149 calories; 3.5 g fat; 20 g carbohydrate; 8.8 g protein

Caribbean Shrimp Salad with Lime Vinaigrette

Cooking time: 25 minutes

Servings: 4

Ingredients:

- 4 cups cooked shrimp, chopped
- 8 cups fresh baby spinach
- 1 cup mango, peeled, chopped
- 1 cup radishes, julienned
- ¼ cup avocado, diced peeled
- ½ cup green onions, sliced
- 5 tablespoons rice vinegar
- 2 tablespoons chili garlic sauce

- 1 ½ tablespoons olive oil
- 1 tablespoon lime zest
- ¼ cup fresh lime juice
- ½ teaspoon paprika
- ½ teaspoon ground cumin
- 2 garlic cloves, minced
- 2 tablespoons unsalted pumpkinseed kernels

Instructions:

1. Mix shrimp, 2 tablespoons vinegar and chili garlic sauce in a bowl, toss well to combine. Cover and refrigerate for 1 hour.

2. Mix the remaining 3 tablespoons vinegar, oil, lemon zest, paprika, cumin, garlic cloves and salt in a bowl, and whisk well.

3. Mix spinach and shrimp mixture in a bowl. Top with mango, radishes and avocado. Serve topped with green onions and pumpkinseed kernels. Drizzle with vinaigrette.

Nutritional info (per serving): 281 calories; 10 g fat; 18.4 g carbohydrate; 30.3 g protein

Grilled Squid Salad with Arugula and Melon

Cooking time: 40 minutes

Servings: 8

Ingredients:

- 1 lb baby squid, cleaned
- 6 anchovy fillets
- ½ teaspoon lemon zest
- ½ teaspoon lime zest
- ½ teaspoon orange zest
- 1 ¼ teaspoons crushed red pepper
- 1 cup extra-virgin olive oil
- 2 cups flat-leaf parsley leaves, chopped
- 4 garlic cloves, smashed

- 2 tablespoons drained capers
- 1 large shallot, chopped
- 2 tablespoons red wine vinegar
- 2 tablespoons lemon juice
- 4 oz baby arugula
- 3 cups cantaloupe cubes
- 2 celery ribs, sliced
- 1 hot red chile, sliced
- Sea salt and freshly ground black pepper, to taste

Instructions:

1. Cut the squid bodies lengthwise, open them.

2. Score a cross-hatch pattern on the insides and transfer to a bowl. Add tentacles, grated citrus zests and 1 teaspoon red-pepper flakes and 1/4 cup of the olive oil, mix well. Cover and refrigerate for 1 hour.

3. Add parsley, anchovies, garlic, capers and shallot to a blender and process until chopped. Add 1/2 cup of the olive oil and pulse to a coarse puree.

4. Add vinegar and the remaining 1/4 teaspoon of crushed red pepper and season with salt and pepper.

5. Preheat grill to medium high. Season squid with salt and grill for about 5 minutes. Slice the squid and transfer to a bowl. Add salsa verde mixture and toss well.

6. Mix the remaining 1/4 cup of olive oil with the lemon juice and season with salt. Add arugula, melon, celery and fresh chile and toss well. Add squid salsa mixture and toss one more time. Serve.

Nutritional info (per serving): 281 calories; 10 g fat; 18.4 g carbohydrate; 30.3 g protein

We can not control everything that comes into our lives
but we can control what goes into our bodies.

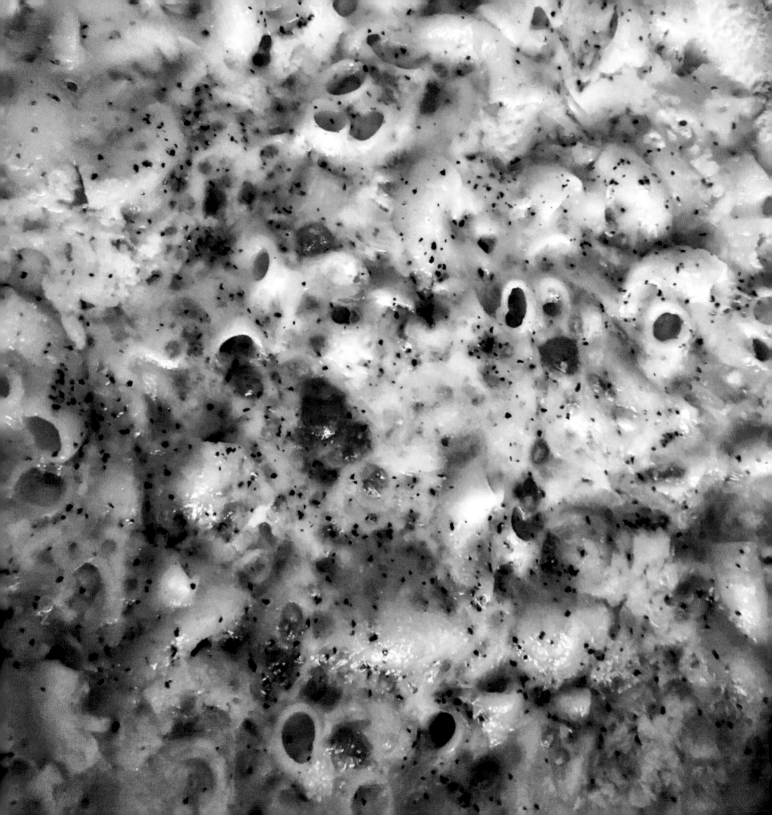

Amiyah's Mac & Cheese

Cooking time: 30 minutes

Servings: 4

Ingredients:

- 8 oz macaroni, cooked
- 3 tablespoons butter, unsalted
- 2 tablespoons flour
- 1 can (12 oz) evaporated milk
- ½ cup half and half
- ½ cup mozzarella cheese, shredded
- ½ cup sharp cheddar cheese, shredded
- ½ cup jack cheese, grated
- 1 tablespoon onion powder
- 2 teaspoons garlic powder
- 1 teaspoon Creole seasoning
- ¼ teaspoon cayenne pepper
- Salt and pepper, to taste

Instructions:

1. Preheat the oven to 375 degrees F.
2. Preheat butter in a skillet over medium heat. Add flour and whisk well to combine, cook for about 1 minute.
3. Add milk and half and half, stir well to combine and simmer for about 4-5 minutes. Season with salt, pepper, onion powder, garlic powder, cayenne and Creole seasoning.
4. Bring to a boil and cook for about 2 minutes. Add mozzarella, cheddar and jack cheese, stir until melted. Add cooked pasta and stir well to combine.
5. Transfer the mixture to the baking dish and bake for 20 minutes.

Nutritional info (per serving): 492 calories; 24 g fat; 47 g carbohydrate; 19 g protein

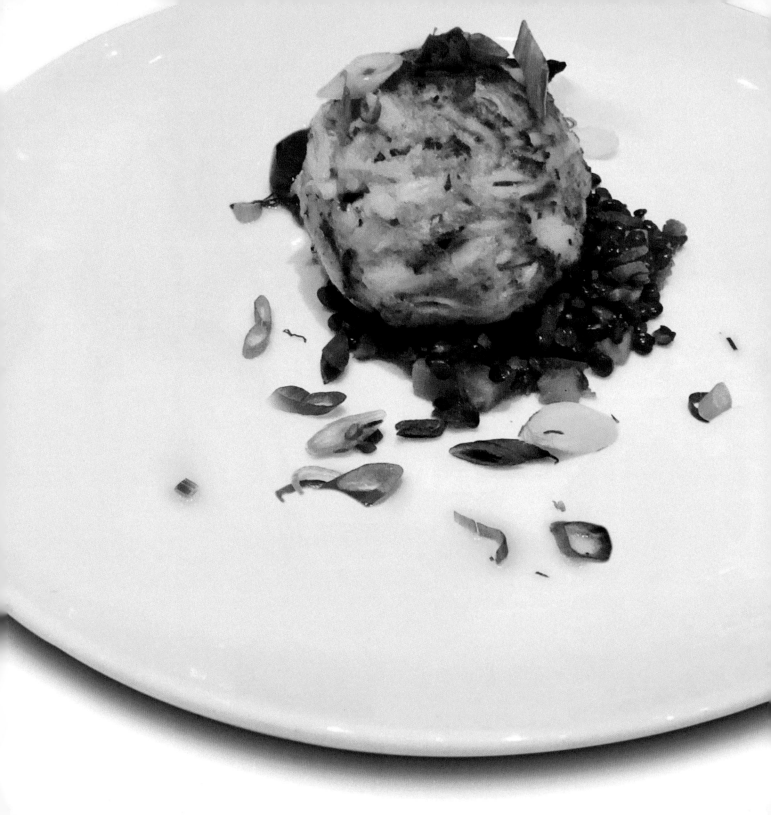

California Crab Cakes

Cooking time: 10 minutes + chilling

Servings: 12

Ingredients:

- 4 cans (6 oz each) crabmeat, drained, flaked
- 4 egg whites
- 1 whole egg
- 2 cups panko bread crumbs
- 6 tablespoons fresh chives, minced
- 3 tablespoons all-purpose flour
- 2 teaspoons hot pepper sauce
- 1 teaspoon baking powder
- ½ teaspoon salt
- ¼ teaspoon pepper
- 2 tablespoons canola oil
- Lemon wedges, for serving

Instructions:

1. Beat the egg and egg whites in a bowl. Add ¾ cup bread crumbs, chives, flour, pepper sauce, baking powder, salt and pepper and mix well to combine.

2. Add crab meat and stir carefully to combine. Cover and refrigerate for at least 2 hours.

3. Add the remaining bread crumbs to a separate shallow bowl. Shape the crab mixture into cakes and dip each cake in breadcrumbs.

4. Preheat oil in a skillet over medium heat. Cook for about 3-4 minutes per side. Serve.

Nutritional info (per serving): 119 calories; 3 g fat; 8 g carbohydrate; 13 g protein

Iceberg Wedges with Shrimp and Blue Cheese Dressing

Cooking time: 15 minutes

Servings: 6

Ingredients:

- 1 ½ lbs large shell-on shrimp
- 3 tablespoons lemon juice
- ½ cup light mayonnaise
- ½ teaspoon hot pepper sauce
- 2 tablespoons blue cheese, crumbled

- 4 tablespoons nonfat milk
- 1 head iceberg lettuce, cut into 12 wedges
- 1 tomato, chopped
- ⅓ cup red onion, sliced

Instructions:

1. Peel and devein shrimp, pat dry with paper towels. Mix shrimp, 2 tablespoons lemon juice and pepper in a bowl, toss well to combine.
2. Mix the remaining 1 tablespoon lemon juice, pepper, mayonnaise and hot sauce in a separate bowl. Add blue cheese and milk, stir well to combine.
3. Preheat grill to medium high heat. Thread the shrimp onto skewers and cook for 3-4 minutes turning once.
4. Top lettuce wedges with shrimp, tomato and onion. Serve with dressing.

Nutritional info (per serving): 190 calories; 10 g fat; 8 g carbohydrate; 18 g protein

Crab Salad with Caesar Vinaigrette

Cooking time: 15 minutes

Servings: 4

Ingredients:

- 8 white anchovies
- 1 lb jumbo lump crabmeat
- ½ lb lettuce leaves
- 1 garlic clove
- 2 tablespoons red wine vinegar
- 1 teaspoon Dijon mustard
- 1 teaspoon Worcestershire sauce

- ¼ cup extra-virgin olive oil
- ¼ cup Parmigiano-Reggiano cheese, grated
- 1 tablespoon snipped chives
- 1 ½ teaspoons tarragon, chopped
- ¼ cup roasted red pepper, diced
- Salt and freshly ground pepper, to taste

Instructions:

1. Add 4 anchovies, garlic, vinegar, mustard and Worcestershire sauce to a blender and process until smooth.
2. Add olive oil and blend until combined. Season with salt and pepper, add Parmesan and blend again.
3. Toss crab, chives, tarragon and red pepper with the vinaigrette. Add romaine and toss well to combine. Top with the remaining anchovies and serve.

Nutritional info (per serving): 285 calories; 18 g fat; 3 g carbohydrate; 12 g protein

Cioppino

Cooking time: 45 minutes

Servings: 6

Ingredients:

- 1 lb large shrimp, shelled and deveined
- 1 lb halibut fillets, cut into 1 ½ inch pieces
- 1 lb king crab leg
- 1 ½ lbs hard-shelled clams, scrubbed
- ¾ lb sea scallops
- 4 garlic cloves, minced
- 2 onions, chopped
- ½ California bay leaf
- 1 teaspoon dried oregano
- 1 teaspoon dried hot red pepper flakes
- ¼ cup olive oil
- 1 bell pepper, diced
- 2 tablespoons tomato paste
- 1 ½ cups dry red wine
- 1 can (32 oz) whole plum tomatoes, chopped
- 1 cup bottled clam juice
- 1 cup chicken broth
- ¼ cup fresh flat-leaf parsley, chopped
- 3 tablespoons fresh basil, chopped
- Salt, pepper, to taste

Instructions:

1. Add garlic, onions, bay leaf, oregano and red pepper flakes to a pot, season with salt and pepper and cook over medium heat for about 5 minutes.

2. Add bell pepper and tomato paste and cook for 1 minute. Add wine and bring to a boil, cook for 5-6 minutes. Add tomatoes with their juices, clam juice and broth and cover the pot. Simmer for about 30 minutes. Season with salt and pepper.

3. Add crab pieces and clams and cook covered for 5-10 minutes. Transfer all opened clams to a plate and discard any unopened ones.

4. Season fish fillets, shrimp and scallops with salt and pepper and simmer covered for about 5 minutes. Discard bay leaves and return clams to pot.

5. Serve topped with parsley.

Nutritional info (per serving): 478 calories; 13 g fat; 20 g carbohydrate; 59 g protein

Cajun Shrimp Salad

Cooking time: 15 minutes

Servings: 5

Ingredients:

- 2 ½ lb shrimp, peeled and deveined
- ¼ cup Italian salad dressing
- 1 tablespoon Cajun seasoning + 1 ½ teaspoon
- 6 oz cream cheese, softened

- ½ cup mayonnaise
- ½ cup celery, chopped
- ¼ cup scallions, chopped
- 1 tablespoon fresh lemon juice
- 1 tablespoon parsley, chopped

Instructions:

1. Mix shrimp, salad dressing and 1 tablespoon Cajun seasoning in a bowl.
2. Preheat a grill pan over medium-high heat and add shrimp. Cook for about 3-4 minutes until cooked, turning once. Transfer to a bowl.
3. Add cream cheese and mayonnaise to a bowl and mix until smooth. Add 1 ½ teaspoon Cajun seasoning, celery, scallions, lemon juice and parsley, and stir well until combined.
4. Add shrimp and toss well to coat. Serve.

Nutritional info (per serving): 250 calories; 13 g fat; 14 g carbohydrate; 26 g protein

It's okay to be a Big fish in a small pan!

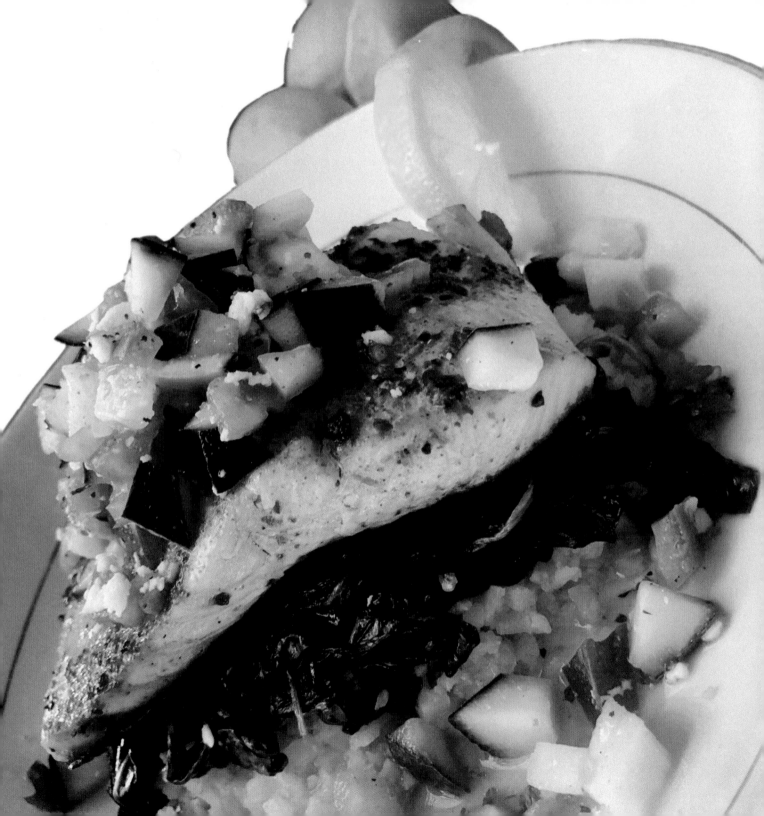

Superwoman Salmon

Prep time: 30 minutes

Servings: 4

Ingredients:

- 2 cups spinach, whilted
- ¼ cup extra-virgin olive oil
- 2 lemons, juiced
- 1 garlic clove, minced
- 1 teaspoon dried oregano
- ½ teaspoon red pepper flakes

- 1 cup feta, cubed
- 1 cup cherry tomatoes, halved
- ¼ cup kalamata olives, sliced
- ¼ cup Persian cucumbers, chopped
- ¼ cup onion, chopped
- 2 tablespoons dill, chopped

For the Salmon:

- 4 salmon fillets
- 1 lemon, thinly sliced

- 1 red onion, sliced
- Salt, pepper, to taste

Instructions:

1. Preheat the oven to 375°F. Mix olive oil, lemon juice, garlic, oregano and red pepper flakes in a bowl. Season with salt and pepper, add feta and toss well to coat. Cover and refrigerate for about 10 minutes.

2. Add sliced lemon and red onion to the baking dish coated with cooking spray. Add salmon fillets, skin side down. Season with salt and pepper and cook for 18-20 minutes.

3. Add tomatoes, olives, cucumbers, chopped red onion and dill to the bowl with Feta. Gently stir to combine.

4. Serve salmon on top of spinach and feta tomatoes salad on top.

Nutritional info (per serving): 385 calories; 16 g fat; 31 g carbohydrate; 37 g protein

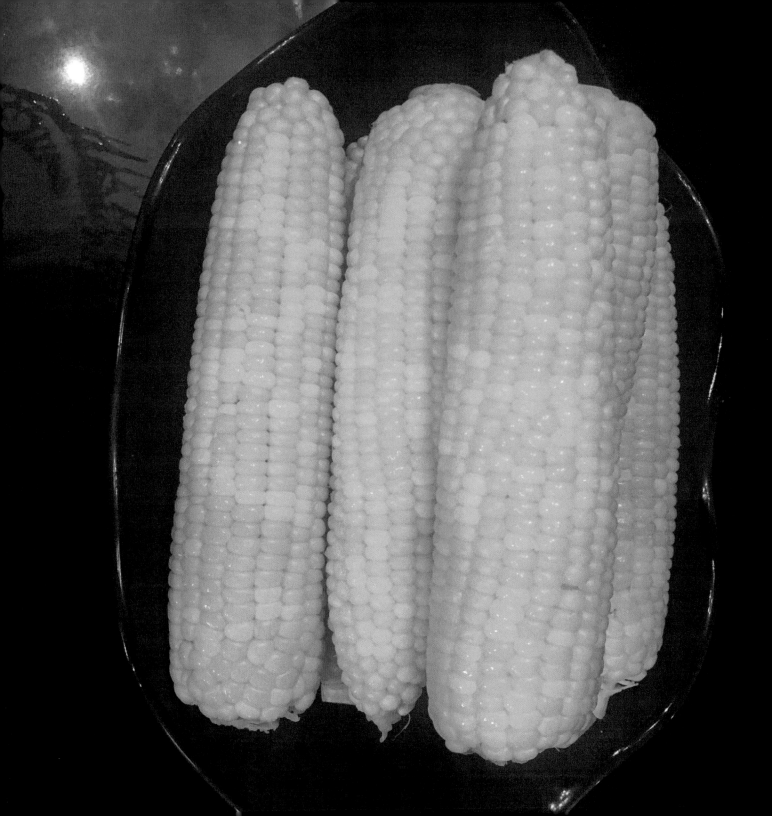

Sweet Southern Corn

Cooking time: 3 hours

Servings: 4

Ingredients:

- 6 ears of corn
- 1 can coconut milk
- 1 stick of butter, cut into pieces
- 2 tablespoons honey

Instructions:

1. Place the corn ears into the pot and cover with milk and water (pour enough to cover the corn).
2. Add butter and honey. Cook for 12-15 minutes. Serve.

Nutritional info (per serving): 146 calories; 3 g fat; 18 g carbohydrate; 11 g protein

Garlic Roasted Salmon with Brussels Sprout

Cooking time: 20 minutes

Servings: 6

Ingredients:

- 2 lbs Brussels sprouts, trimmed
- 6 salmon fillets, skin removed
- Olive oil
- 4 garlic cloves, minced
- 1 tablespoon dried oregano
- 1 lemon, sliced
- Salt, black pepper, to taste

Instructions:

1. Preheat the oven to 450F. Grease a baking sheet with cooking spray.
2. Mix Brussels sprouts, about 3 tablespoons olive oil, salt and pepper in a bowl. Spread the sprouts onto the baking sheet and cook for 15 minutes. Stir once while cooking.
3. Drizzle salmon fillets with olive oil, season with oregano, salt and pepper, divide garlic among all fillets.
4. Place salmon on top of cooked sprouts and bake for 10-12 minutes. Serve topped with lemon slices.

Nutritional info (per serving): 334 calories; 15 g fat; 10 g carbohydrate; 33 g protein

The only possession we truly have is our bodies, give it the care it deserves.

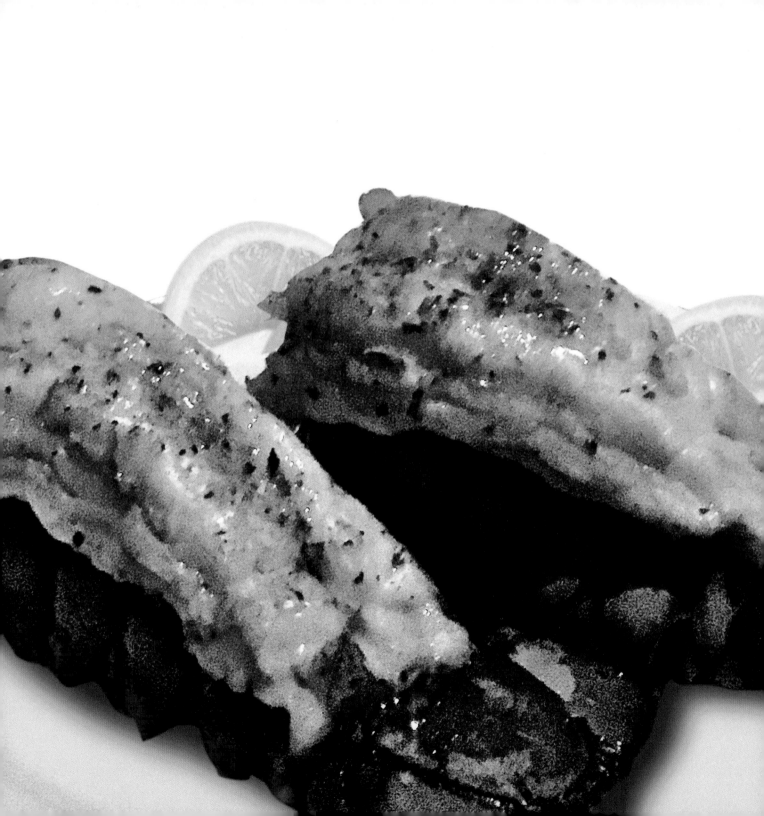

Cajun Lobster Tails

Cooking time: 10 minutes

Servings: 2

Ingredients:

- 2 lobster tails, snipped through the top of the shell and cut through part of the meat
- 2 tablespoons butter, melted + 1 tablespoon
- 2 tablespoons lemon juice
- 1 garlic clove, minced
- 2 tablespoons bread crumbs
- 2 tablespoons Parmesan cheese, grated
- 1 teaspoon Cajun seasoning
- 1 teaspoon paprika
- Salt, to taste
- Chopped fresh parsley, for serving

Instructions:

1. Carefully pry open the shell of each lobster tail wide enough to separate the meat from the shell. Leave the attached tail.
2. Mix 2 tablespoons butter, lemon juice and garlic in a bowl. Brush each lobster tail with the mixture, coat well.
3. Preheat the broiler. Broil the lobster tails for about 10 minutes.
4. Mix breadcrumbs, Parmesan, 1 tablespoon butter, Cajun seasoning, paprika and salt in a bowl.
5. Remove the lobster tails from the oven and top with bread crumb mixture. Return to the broiler and cook for 1-2 minutes. Serve topped with parsley.

Nutritional info (per serving): 234 calories; 10.5 g fat; 14 g carbohydrate; 20 g protein

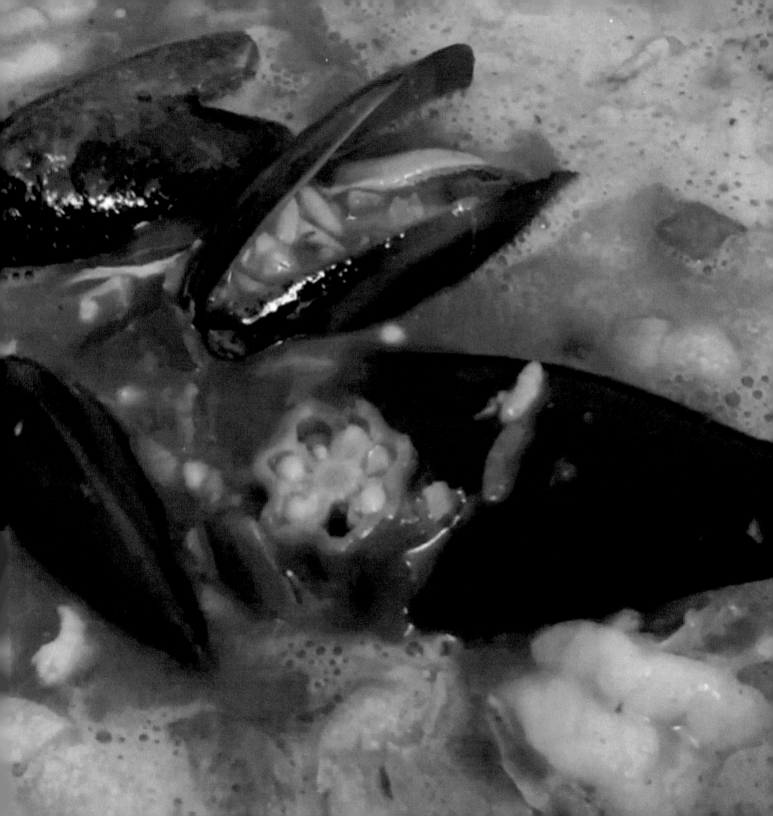

Grannie's Gumbo

Cooking time: 2 hours

Servings: 10

Ingredients:

- 1 lb mussels
- 1 ½ lbs medium shrimp, peeled and deveined
- 1 lb lump crabmeat
- 1 package (10 oz) frozen cut okra, thawed
- ½ lb andouille sausage, sliced
- 2 tablespoons butter
- ½ can tomato sauce
- ½ can stewed tomatoes
- ½ cup flour
- ½ cup celery, chopped
- ½ onion, chopped

- 1 bell pepper, chopped
- 1 garlic clove, minced
- 1 ½ quarts water
- 3 cubes vegetable bouillon
- 1 tablespoon hot pepper sauce
- ½ tablespoon white sugar
- ¼ teaspoon Cajun seasoning
- 2 bay leaves
- ¼ teaspoon dried thyme leaves
- 1 teaspoon gumbo file powder
- 1 tablespoon white vinegar
- 1 tablespoon Worcestershire sauce

Instructions:

1. Add celery, onions,bell pepper, and garlic to food processor and pulse until finely chopped or chop by hand.
2. Whisk flour and butter in a heavy saucepan over medium-low heat until paste forms. Add vegetables and sausage, and stir well.
3. Add more water and bring the mixture to a simmer over medium-low heat, cook for about 10-15 minutes.

4. Add the remaining water and vegetable bouillon cubes to a pot and bring to a boil. Stir until the bouillon cubes dissolve, add vegetables and reduce the heat to low. Add sugar, salt, hot pepper sauce, Cajun seasoning, bay leaves, thyme, stewed tomatoes and tomato sauce.

5. Cook over low heat for 1 hour. After about 45 minutes add gumbo powder.

6. Melt more butter in a skillet and add okra and vinegar, cook for 15 minutes. Add the mixture into the gumbo. Add crab meat, mussels and worcestershire sauce, simmer for about 45. Add Shrimp the last 8 min. If mussels don't open disgard. Serve as is or enjoy over rice.

Nutritional info (per serving): 296 calories; 17.9 g fat; 12.1 g carbohydrate; 20.9 g protein

Go eat your food with gladness and drink your wine with a joyful heart, for God has already approved what you do-Ecclesiastes 9:7

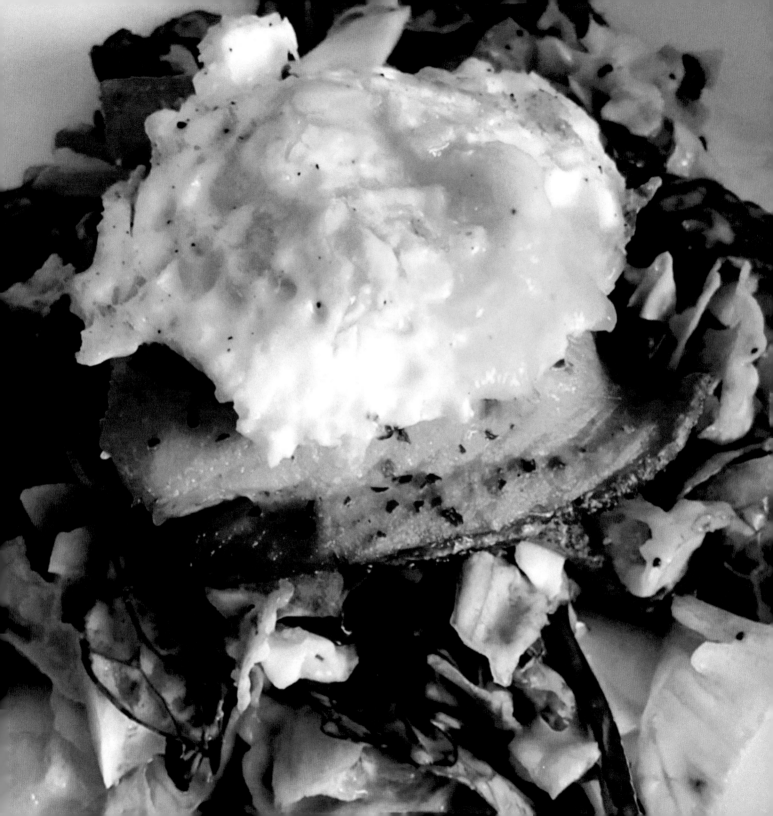

Roasted Salmon with Salad and Egg

Cooking time: 25 minutes

Servings: 4

Ingredients:

- 4 salmon fillets
- 1 packet green mix
- 6tablespoons olive oil
- 2 tablespoons soy sauce
- 1 teaspoon Dijon mustard
- 1 teaspoon lemon juice and zest
- 1 egg, fried
- Salt, pepper, to taste

Instructions:

1. Preheat the oven to 450 F.
2. Mix soy sauce, Dijon mustard, lemon juice and zest in a bowl.
3. Toss greens with olive oil, salt and pepper. Pour the soy sauce mixture on top of greens.
4. Season salmon with salt and pepper and place on the baking sheet. Bake for 10 minutes.
5. Serve salmon on top of greens and egg. Serve.

Nutritional info (per serving): 145 calories; 9 g fat; 8 g carbohydrate; 11 g protein

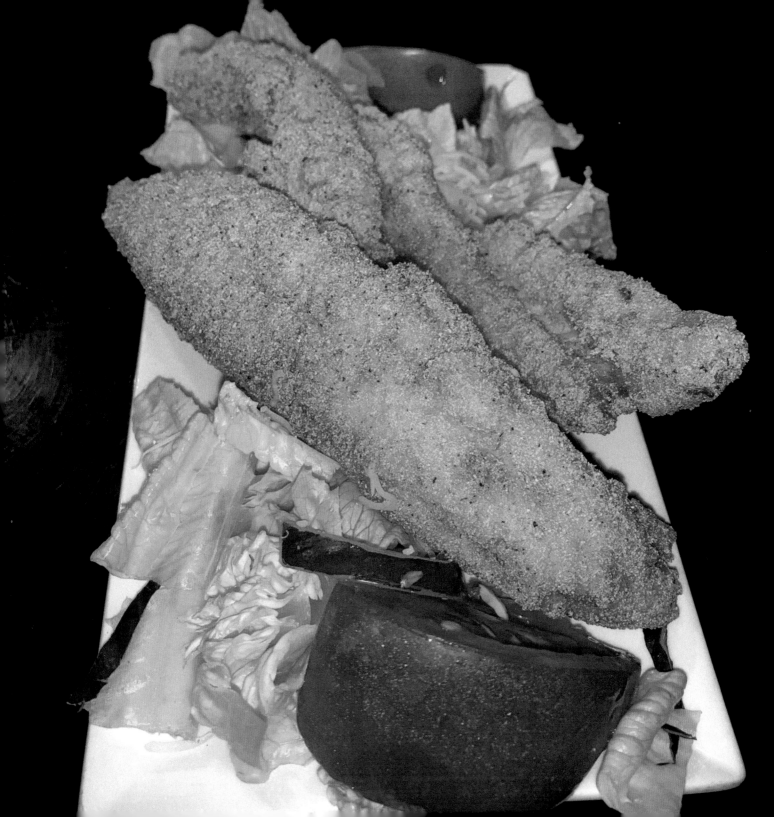

Southern Fried Catfish

Cooking time: 15 minutes

Servings: 4

Ingredients:

- 4 catfish fillets
- 1 ½ cup cornmeal
- 1 tablespoon garlic powder
- 1 teaspoons onion powder
- 1 teaspoon cayenne pepper

- 1 teaspoon white pepper
- 1 ½ cups buttermilk
- Oil for frying
- Salt, to taste

Instructions:

1. Preheat oil in a deep fryer until 375 F.
2. Mix cornmeal, garlic, onion powder, cayenne, salt and pepper in a bowl. Dip each fish fillet first in buttermilk and then into cornmeal mixture.
3. Add to the deep fryer and cook for about 3-4 minutes per side. Transfer to a plate lined with paper towel. Serve.

Nutritional info (per serving): 146 calories; 3 g fat; 18 g carbohydrate; 11 g protein

Salmon Foil Packets with Vegetables

Cooking time: 15 minutes

Servings: 4

Ingredients:

- 1 ½ lbs (680 g) salmon fillets
- ½ lb (225 g) asparagus, trimmed, halved
- 10 oz (280 g) grape tomatoes
- 10 oz (280 g) zucchini, sliced
- ¼ cup (65 ml) olive oil

- ½ lemon, juiced and zested
- 2 garlic cloves, minced
- 1 tablespoon (14 g) fresh parsley, chopped
- 1 tablespoon (14 g) fresh dill, chopped
- Salt, pepper, to taste

Instructions:

1. Preheat the oven to 400 F.
2. Prepare 4 squares of foil. Place salmon fillets in the center of each piece of foil. Add asparagus, tomatoes and zucchini next to the fillets.
3. Mix olive oil, salt, pepper, lemon juice, lemon zest, minced garlic, parsley and dill in a bowl.
4. Pour the mixture on top of each fillet and over veggies. Fold the foil and seal. Place on the baking sheet and bake for 15-20 minutes. Serve.

Nutritional info (per serving): 400 calories; 24 g fat; 8 g total carbs; 6 g net carbs; 36 g protein

They say you are what you eat, just call me fish!

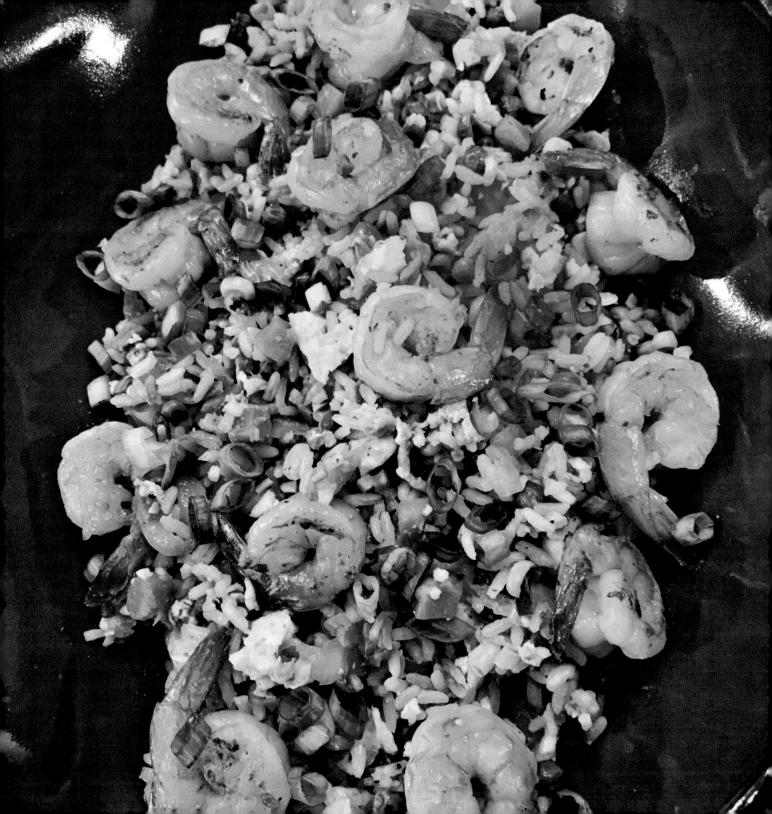

Shrimp Fried Rice

Cooking time: 15 minutes

Servings: 4

Ingredients:

- 4 cups rice, cooked
- 8 oz raw shrimp, shelled and deveined
- ½ teaspoon cornstarch
- 3 tablespoons canola oil
- 3 eggs, beaten
- 2 stalks green onion, minced
- ¾ cup frozen peas and carrots
- 1 tablespoon soy sauce
- 1 teaspoon dark toasted sesame oil

Instructions:

1. Sprinkle shrimp with salt, pepper and cornstarch. Preheat oil in a pan over medium heat. Add shrimp and cook for about 1 minute per side. Transfer to a plate.
2. Add eggs to the skillet and cook until done, stirring often. Transfer to a plate.
3. Add green onions and rice, stir well to combine. Add the remaining ingredients and stir well for 1-2 minutes. Serve

Nutritional info (per serving): 335 calories; 12 g fat; 12 g carbohydrate; 15 g protein

Lobster Mashed Potatoes

Cooking time: 25 minutes

Servings: 8

Ingredients:

- 6 Yukon Gold potatoes, peeled and quartered
- 3 tablespoons unsalted butter
- 2 garlic cloves, minced
- ½ cup whole milk
- 2 tablespoons full-fat cream cheese
- 1 cup lobster chunks, cooked
- ½ cup Cheddar cheese, grated
- 2 tablespoons fresh chives, chopped
- Sea salt and pepper, to taste

Instructions:

1. Add potatoes to a large pot and cover with water. Bring to a boil and reduce the heat to low, cook for 20-25 minutes.
2. Melt butter in a sauce pan over medium heat. Add garlic and cook for about 45 seconds, stirring constantly.
3. Drain potatoes and reserve about 1 cup water. Mash potatoes adding potatoes cooking water. Add garlic butter mixture, milk, cream cheese, salt and pepper and mash well until fluffy and smooth.
4. Add lobster cheddar and chives, stir well and serve.

Nutritional info (per serving): 214 calories; 9 g fat; 27 g carbohydrate; 8 g protein

*If you require a healthy body than you are
required to eat healthy foods*

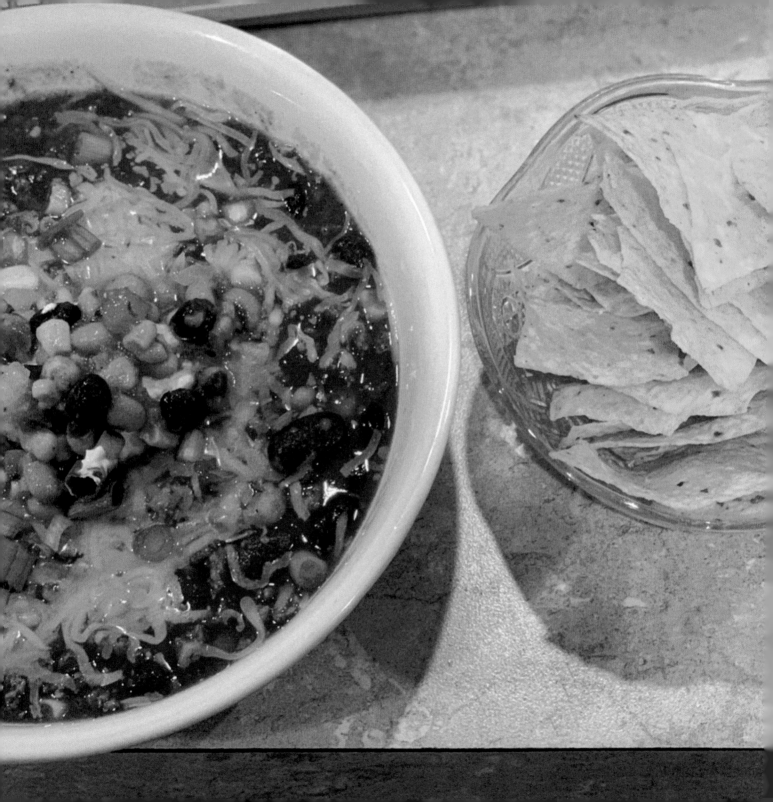

Shay's Vegetarian Chili

Cooking time: 40 minutes

Servings: 4

Ingredients:

- 1 red onion, chopped
- 1 bell pepper, chopped
- 2 carrots, chopped
- 2 celery ribs, chopped
- 1 can (28 oz) diced tomatoes, undrained
- 2 cans (15 oz each) black beans, rinsed and drained
- 1 can (15 oz) pinto beans, rinsed and drained
- 2 tablespoons olive oil
- 4 garlic cloves, minced

- 2 teaspoons chili powder
- 2 teaspoons ground cumin
- 1 ½ teaspoons smoked paprika
- 1 teaspoon dried oregano
- 1 bay leaf
- 2 cups vegetable broth
- 2 teaspoons red wine vinegar
- 2 tablespoons fresh cilantro, chopped
- Salt, pepper, to taste
- Shredded cheese, for serving

Instructions:

1. Preheat oil in a pot over medium heat. Add onion, carrot, bell pepper, celery, salt and pepper. Cook for about 8-10 minutes, stirring often.
2. Add garlic, chili powder, cumin, paprika and oregano. Cook for 1 minute more.
3. Add tomatoes, all the beans, bay leaf, vinegar and broth, bring everything to a boil. Reduce the heat and cook chili for 30 minutes.
4. Adjust seasoning to taste and serve topped with cheese and cilantro.

Nutritional info (per serving): 389 calories; 24 g fat; 25 g carbohydrate; 56 g protein

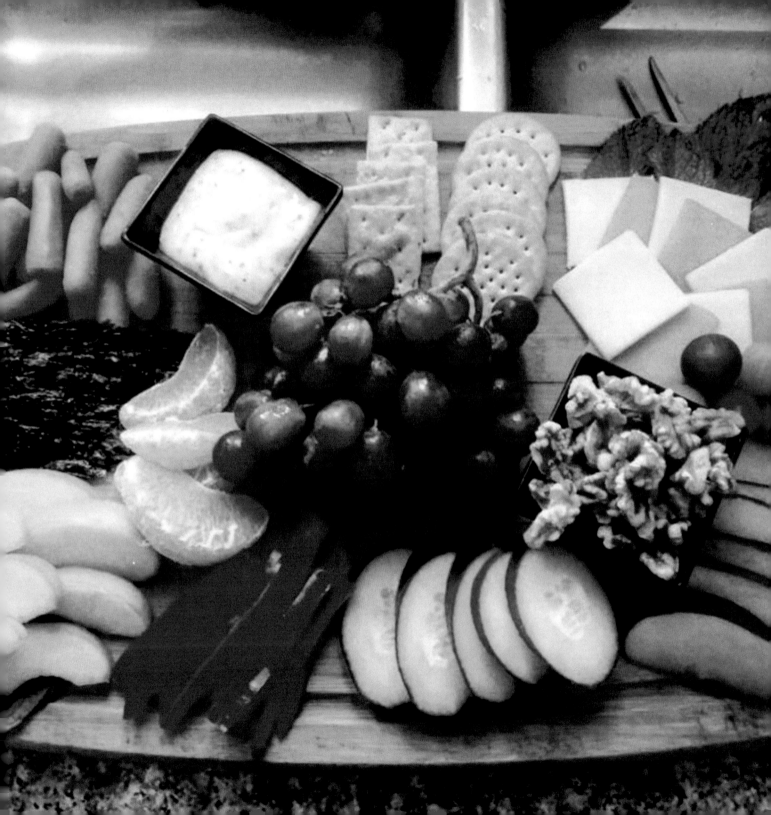

Trophy Model delight

Cooking time: 5 minutes

Servings: 4

Ingredients:

- Baby carrots
- Grapes
- 2 apples, slices
- 1 bell pepper, sliced
- Crackers

- Cheese slices
- 1 cucumber, sliced
- 1 mandarin orange
- 1 cup walnuts
- Ranch dressing

Instructions:

1. Arrange everything on a tray or a platter. Serve.

Nutritional info (per serving): 150 calories; 8 g fat; 23 g carbohydrate; 6 g protein

Shrimp Cobb Salad with Cilantro Lime Vinaigrette

Cooking time: 20 minutes

Servings: 2

Ingredients:

- 1 lb shrimp, peeled and deveined
- 2 tablespoons olive oil
- 1 tablespoon Creole seasoning
- 4 slices bacon, diced
- 2 eggs, hard boiled, halved

- 5 cups romaine lettuce, chopped
- 1 avocado, diced
- 1 cup canned corn kernels, drained
- ½ cup goat cheese, crumbled

For the Dressing:

- 1 cup loosely packed cilantro, stems removed
- 1 lime, juiced
- 1 jalapeño, chopped

- 2 garlic cloves
- 2 tablespoons olive oil
- 2 tablespoons apple cider vinegar
- Salt, pepper, to taste

Instructions:

1. Mix cilantro, lime juice, jalapeño and garlic in a bowl, season with salt and pepper. Add olive oil and vinegar and whisk well to combine.

2. Preheat the oven to 400F. Prepare a baking sheet and line it with parchment paper. Place shrimp on the tray and bake for 4-5 minutes.

3. Preheat skillet over medium heat and add bacon, cook until crispy, for 6-8 minutes. Transfer to a plate.

4. Place lettuce to a bowl, top with rows of shrimp, bacon, eggs, avocado, corn and goat cheese. Serve topped with cilantro lime vinaigrette.

Nutritional info (per serving): 270 calories; 15 g fat; 12 g carbohydrate; 23 g protein

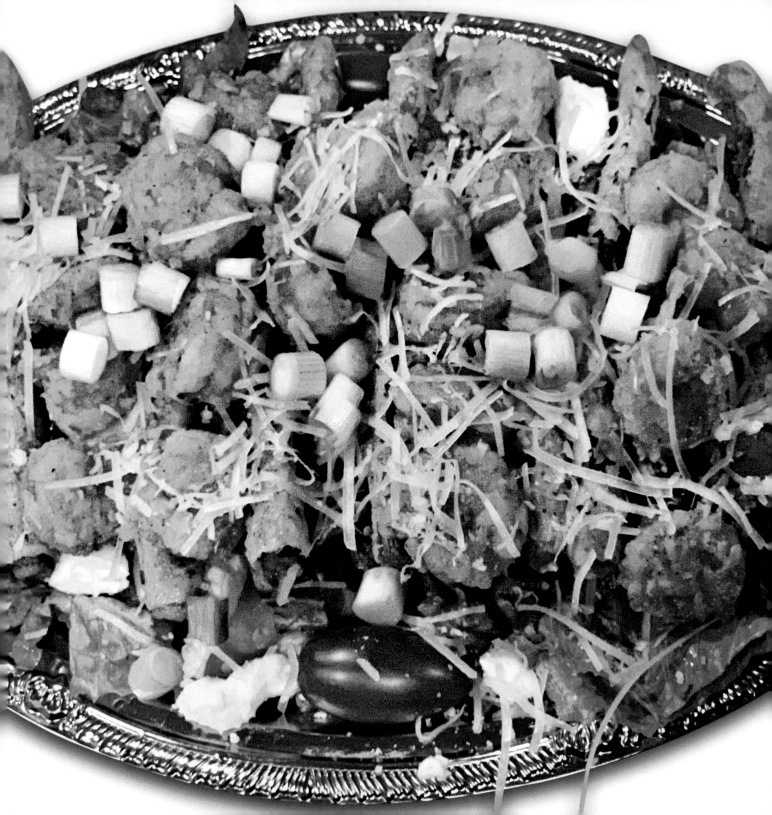

Tempura Shrimp Salad

Cooking time: 10 minutes

Servings: 4

Ingredients:

- 1 lb unpeeled, large shrimp
- 1 lb asparagus
- 1 cup tempura batter mix
- ¾ cup cold light beer
- 2 teaspoons fajita seasoning mix
- Lettuce, chopped
- 1 cup grape tomatoes
- Green onions, chopped
- Vegetable oil, for frying

Instructions:

1. Mix tempura batter mix, beer, and seasoning in a bowl; let rest for 5 minutes.
2. Preheat oil in a deep pan over medium heat. Dip each shrimp and asparagus into the batter mix and cook for 1-2 minutes per side.
3. Place the lettuce leaves on the plate. Top with asparagus and shrimp. Top with tomatoes and green onions. Serve.

Nutritional info (per serving): 254 calories; 18 g fat; 13 g carbohydrate; 18 g protein

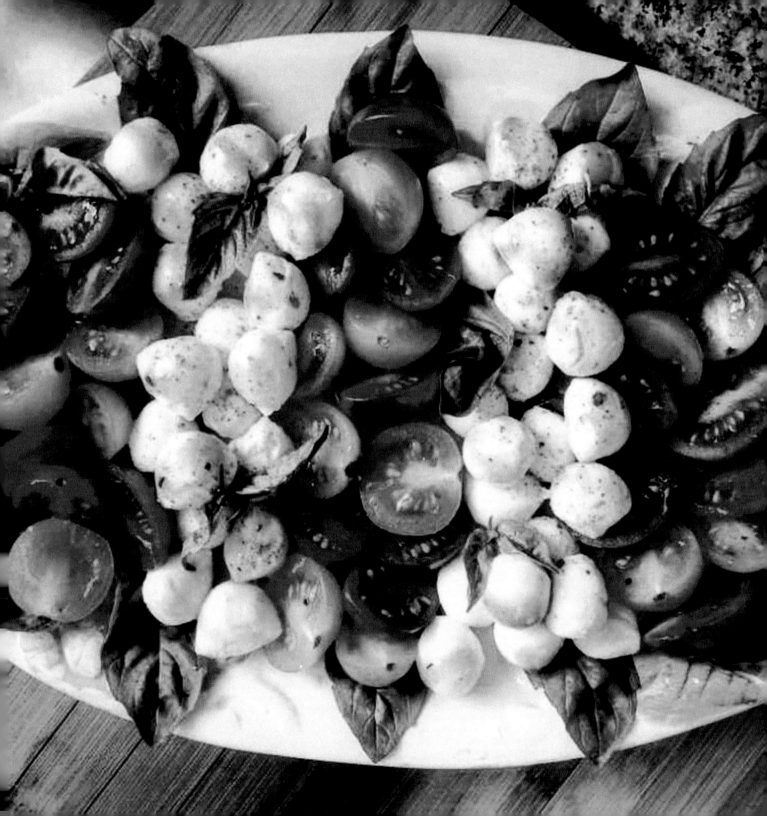

Heirloom Tomato Caprese Salad

Cooking time: 5 minutes

Servings: 4

Ingredients:

- 1 pint cherry heirloom tomatoes, halved
- 8 oz mozzarella balls
- ¼ cup extra virgin olive oil
- ¼ cup balsamic vinegar
- 1 tablespoon fresh basil leaves
- Salt, pepper, to taste

Instructions:

1. Mix oil, balsamic vinegar, salt and pepper in a bowl.
2. Place the tomatoes, basil leaves, mozzarella on a platter and drizzle with the oil mixture. Serve.

Nutritional info (per serving): 202 calories; 6 g fat; 13 g carbohydrate; 16 g protein

Pan-Fried Sea Bass with Tomato and Basil

Cooking time: 30 minutes

Servings: 6

Ingredients:

- 6 whole sea bass fillets
- ½ cup olive oil
- 2 shallots, chopped
- 1 lb cherry tomatoes, halved

- 6 sprigs basil, chopped
- 1 cup rocket
- ¼ cup reduced balsamic vinegar
- Salt, pepper, to taste

Instructions:

1. Preheat oil in a pan over medium heat. Add shallots and salt, cook for 2-3 minutes. Add tomatoes and cook for 2-3 minutes more. Add basil, stir well and remove from the heat.
2. Preheat oil in a separate pan and add fish. Cook for 2 minutes per side until golden brown. Season with salt and pepper.
3. Serve browned fish with cooked tomatoes and rocket leaves, drizzle with oil and top with balsamic vinegar.

Nutritional info (per serving): 341 calories; 26.2 g fat; 5.1 g carbohydrate; 23.1 g protein

In my house, a man who doesn't cook doesn't eat-Rhea

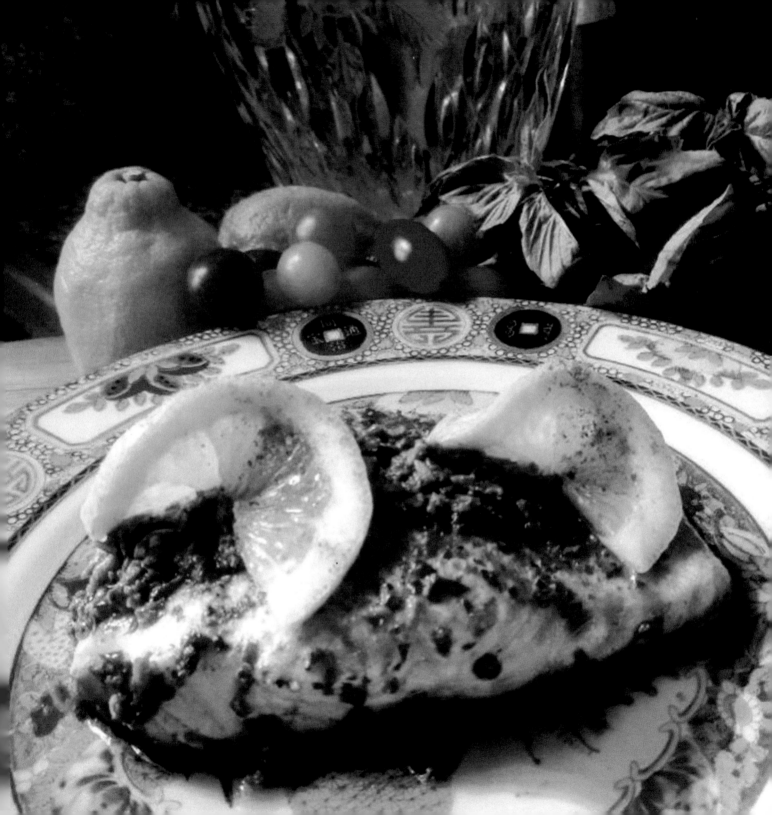

Pesto Salmon

Cook time: 25 minutes

Servings: 4

Ingredients:

- 2 lbs salmon fillets
- 2 oz green pesto + 2 oz
- 1 cup mayonnaise
- ½ cup dairy free yogurt
- Salt, pepper, to taste

Instructions:

1. Preheat the oven to 400F. Prepare a baking dish and spray it with cooking spray.
2. Place the salmon in the baking dish and spread 2 oz pesto on top of each fillet. Season with salt and pepper.
3. Bake for about 25 minutes. Mix 2 oz pesto, mayo and yogurt in a bowl and serve cooked salmon with the sauce.

Nutritional info (per serving): 684 calories; 52.4 g fat; 2 g total carbs; 2 g net carbs; 39.7 g protein

Salmon Croquettes

Cook time: 15 minutes

Servings: 12

Ingredients:

- 1 can (15 ½ oz) pink salmon, drained and flaked
- 3 eggs, beaten
- 1 ½ cups crackers, crushed
- ½ teaspoon salt
- ¼ teaspoon red pepper
- Vegetable oil

Instructions:

1. Mix salmon, eggs, cracker crumbs, salt and pepper in a bowl and mix well to combine.
2. Shape the mixture into 12 croquettes. Preheat oil in a skillet over medium heat. Fry the croquettes until golden brown. Drain on paper towels and serve.

Nutritional info (per serving): 225 calories; 11.9 g fat; 15 g total carbs; 14.6 g protein

*You don't really need to cook well, you just need
to add a special ingredient, Love!*

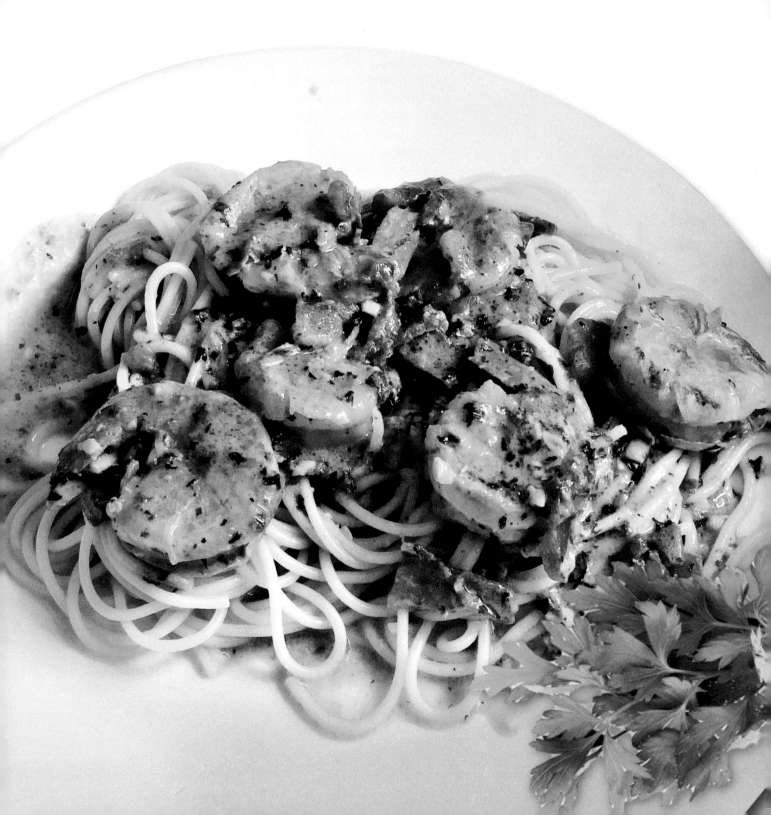

Shrimp Scampi

Cooking time: 10 minutes

Servings: 2

Ingredients:

- 1 lb shrimp, deveined
- 12 oz spaghetti, cooked
- 2 tablespoons ghee
- ¼ cup chicken broth
- 2 tablespoons lemon juice
- 2 tablespoons parsley, chopped
- A pinch red chili flakes
- Salt, pepper, to taste

Instructions:

1. Preheat a skillet over medium heat and add ghee, melt. Add chicken broth, lemon juice and red chili flakes, bring everything to a boil and add shrimp.
2. Simmer for about 5-8 minutes and reduce the heat to low.
3. Season with salt and pepper to taste, add pasta and parsley, toss well to coat. Serve.

Nutritional info (per serving): 366 calories; 15 g fat; 7 g total carbs; 5 g net carbs; 49 g protein

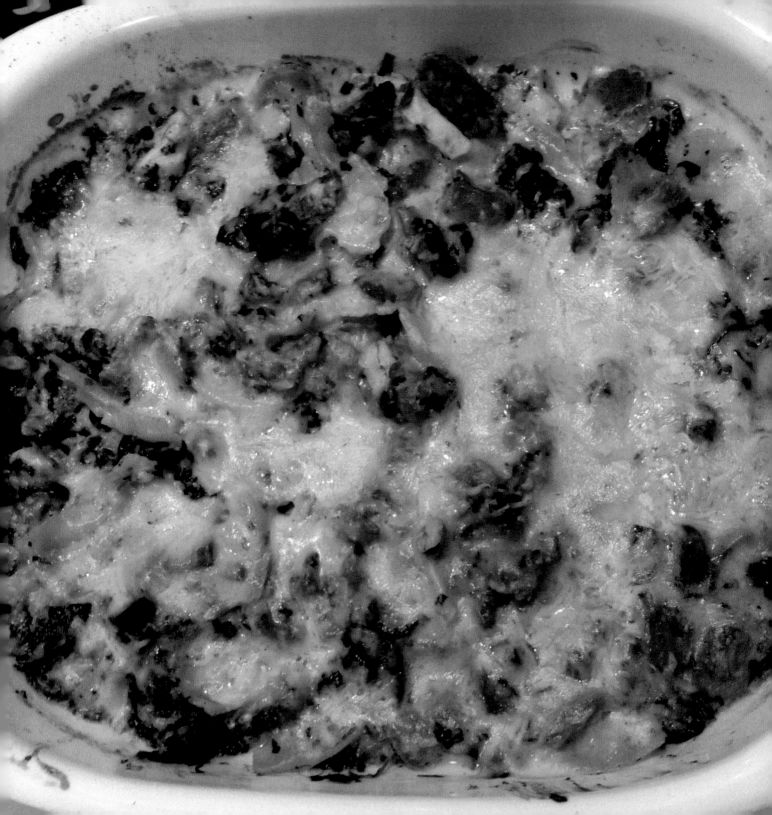

Tessa's Tuna Noodle Casserole

Cook time: 25 minutes

Servings: 4

Ingredients:

- 8 oz egg noodles, cooked and drained
- 2 cans (3 oz each) tuna packed in oil, drained
- ⅓ cup bread crumbs
- 3 tablespoons unsalted butter
- 3 tablespoons all-purpose flour

- 1 cup low-fat milk
- 1 cup spinach
- 1 cup low-sodium chicken broth
- ½ cup Cheddar cheese, shredded
- 2 tablespoons vegetable oil
- Salt and pepper, to taste

Instructions:

1. Preheat the oven to 375°F. Prepare a baking dish and grease it with cooking spray.
2. Melt butter in a pan over medium-high heat. Add flour and cook for 2 minutes. Whisk in milk and broth. Cook for about 10 minutes, stirring all the time. Season with salt and pepper.
3. Mix noodles,sauce, tuna, spinach   and spread in baking dish.
4. Mix bread crumbs and cheese in a bowl. Sprinkle over baking dish and drizzle with olive oil. Bake for 20-25 minutes.

Nutritional info (per serving): 633 calories; 29 g fat; 33 g total carbs; 29 g protein

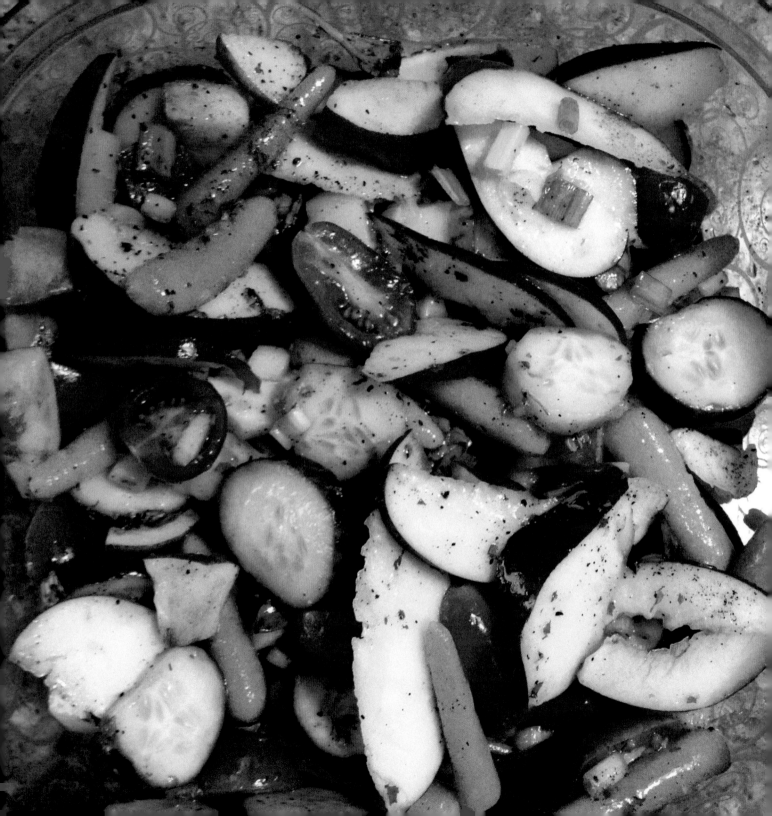

Summer Breeze Salad

Cook time: 5 minutes

Servings: 4

Ingredients:

- 3 ½ oz baby carrots
- 1 cucumber, sliced
- 1 apple, sliced
- 1 cup grape tomatoes, halved
- ¼ cup green onions, chopped
- 2 tablespoons cilantro, chopped
- ¼ cup olive oil
- Salt, pepper, to taste

Instructions:

1. Mix all ingredients in a bowl. Season with salt and pepper and toss well to coat. Serve.

Nutritional info (per serving): 115 calories; 6 g fat; 15 g total carbs; 3 g protein

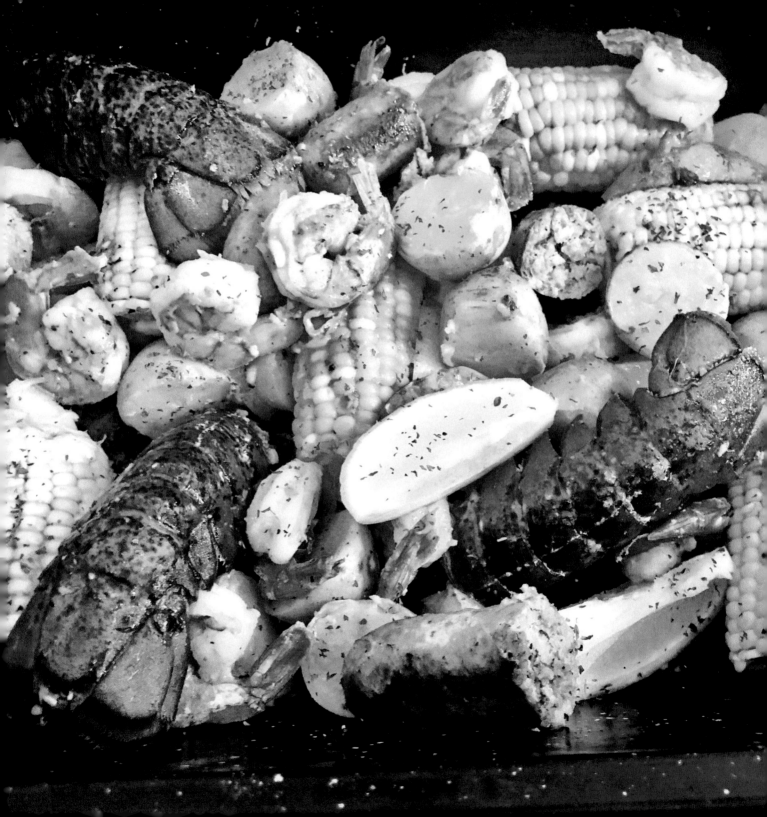

Brae's Seafood Boil

Cooking time: 10 minutes

Servings: 4

Ingredients:

- 1lb Shrimp shell-on
- 8 andouille sausages, sliced
- 8 red potatoes, halved
- 4 onions, quartered
- 2 ears corn, cut in halves
- 4 lobster tails
- ½ cup seafood seasoning

Instructions:

1. Bring a pot of water to a boil. Add potatoes and cook for 20 minutes.
2. Add the remaining ingredients, except shrimp and cook for 10 minutes more. Add Shrimp and cook for 5 minutes than turn heat off.
3. Drain everything and sprinkle on preferred seafood seasoning. add lemon slices as garnish. Serve on a large platter.

Nutritional info (per serving): 416 calories; 11.1 g fat; 46.2 g carbohydrate; 34.1 g protein

Happy Butter Sauce

Ingredients:

- 2 sticks of unsalted butter
- juice of two lemons
- 1/4 cup of minced garlic
- 2 tbsp of cajun seasonings* 1tsp lemon pepper
- 1/2 tsp cayenne pepper, optional.

Instruction:

1. Melt butter in sauce pan, stir in all other ingredients.
2. Cook for about 7 minutes.enjoy by pouring over entire boil or use as a dipping sauce.

Scallop Piccata

Cook time: 30 minutes

Servings: 4

Ingredients:

- 1 ½ lbs sea scallops
- 1 package (10 oz) fresh baby spinach
- 5 teaspoons canola oil
- 1 garlic clove, chopped
- ½ cup vermouth

- 3 tablespoons fresh parsley, chopped
- 2 tablespoons fresh lemon juice
- 2 tablespoons butter
- 4 teaspoons capers
- Salt, pepper, to taste

Instructions:

1. Preheat a skillet over high heat. Pat scallops dry with paper towels and sprinkle with salt and pepper. Add 1 tablespoon canola oil to the pan and add scallops, cook for about 2 minutes per side. Remove from the pan.

2. Reduce the heat to medium and add chopped garlic, cook for about 10 seconds. Add vermouth and cook for 2 minutes. Remove from heat and add parsley, fresh lemon juice, butter and capers, stir until butter melts. Transfer the sauce to a bowl.

3. Preheat the remaining 2 teaspoons oil in pan over medium-high heat. Add spinach and sauté for about 30 seconds. Drizzle sauce over scallops and serve with spinach.

Nutritional info (per serving): 275 calories; 13.1 g fat; 8.3 g total carbs; 30.9 g protein

Kind words are like honeycomb, sweet to the soul and healthy for the body- Proverb 16:24

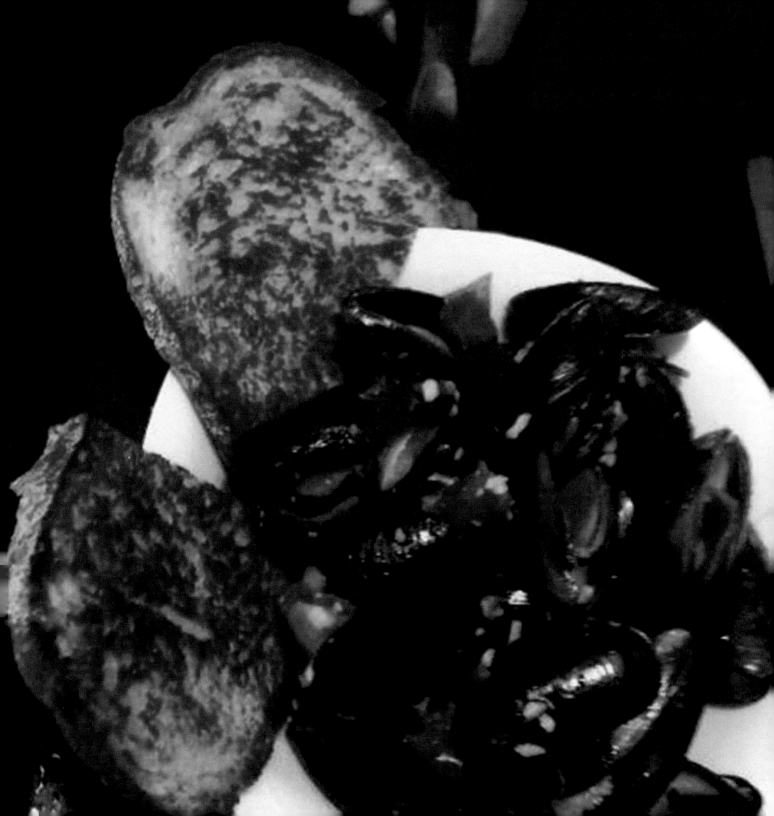

Mighty Mussels

Cook time: 30 minutes

Servings: 2

Ingredients:

- 1 can (14.5 oz) no salt-added stewed tomatoes, undrained and chopped
- 1 bottle (8 oz) clam juice
- 2 lbs small mussels, scrubbed and debearded
- 2 teaspoons olive oil

- 2 teaspoons garlic, minced
- ¼ cup dry white wine
- 1 teaspoon fresh lemon juice
- ¼ teaspoon crushed red pepper
- 2 tablespoons fresh flat-leaf parsley, chopped

Instructions:

1. Preheat oil in a pan over medium heat. Add garlic and cook for about 1 minute. Add wine, lemon juice, pepper, tomatoes, and clam juice and bring everything to a boil.

2. Add mussels and cover the pan, reduce the heat to low and cook for 5 minutes until shells open.

3. Remove from heat and discard any unopened shells. Serve topped with parsley.

Nutritional info (per serving): 295 calories; 8.9 g fat; 21.4 g total carbs; 25.4 g protein

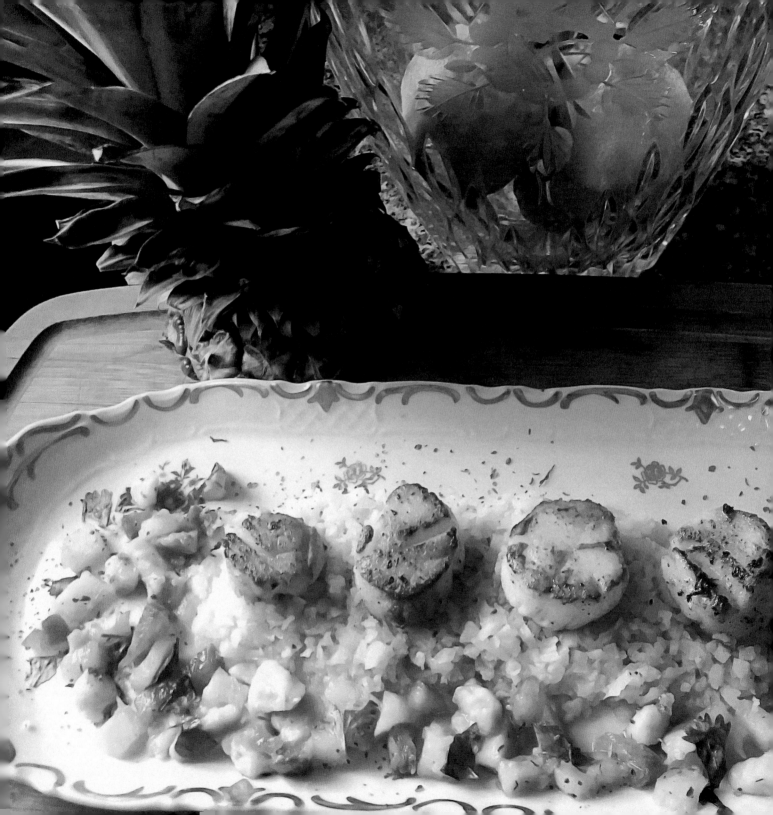

Scallops with Avocado and Pineapple Salsa

Cook time: 7 minutes

Servings: 2

Ingredients:

- 5-6 sea scallops
- 2 cups pineapple chunks
- ½ cup red onion, chopped
- 1 avocado, peeled, pitted and cubed
- ⅓ cup fresh cilantro, chopped
- 2 tablespoons lime juice

- 2 tablespoons olive oil
- ½ tablespoon lemon juice
- 1 tablespoon butter, cubed
- 2 cups rice, cooked
- Salt and pepper, to taste

Instructions:

1. Mix pineapple, onion, avocado, cilantro and lime juice in a bowl. Toss well to coat.
2. Rinse and pat dry the scallops. Season with salt and pepper, preheat oil in a pan over medium heat.
3. Add scallops and cook for 2-3 minutes per side. Serve scallops on top of rice with pineapple salad.

Nutritional info (per serving): 135 calories; 11 g fat; 22 g total carbs; 15 g protein

Creole Fish Stew

Cooking time: 45 minutes

Servings: 4

Ingredients:

- 1 ½ lbs cod fillet, cut into 2-inch pieces
- ½ cup long-grain white rice
- 1 can (14.5 oz) diced tomatoes
- ⅓ cup canola oil
- ⅓ cup all-purpose flour
- 1 cup yellow onion, chopped
- 1 bell pepper, chopped
- 1 cup celery, chopped
- 3 garlic cloves, minced
- 1 ½ teaspoon paprika
- ½ teaspoon dried thyme
- 1 bay leaf
- 1 cup water
- 2 cups chicken broth
- 2 green onions, chopped
- 2 tablespoons fresh parsley, chopped
- A pinch cayenne pepper
- Salt, pepper, to taste

Instructions:

1. Preheat the oven to 350 F. Preheat oil in a skillet over medium heat. Add flour and stir well, cook for 10-15 minutes, stirring constantly.
2. Add onion, bell peppers and celery and cook for 5-7 minutes. Add garlic, paprika, thyme, bay leaf, and cayenne and cook for 2 more minutes. Add tomatoes, water and chicken broth and bring everything to a boil.
3. Add rice, cover the pot and place into the oven. Bake for 25 minutes.
4. Season fish with salt and pepper. Remove the pot from the oven and add fish to the pot. Cover and return to the oven for 5-7 minutes. Add sliced green onions and chopped parsley and serve.

Nutritional info (per serving): 467 calories; 20.3 g fat; 11.6 g total carbs; 31 g protein

In my parents house, mama has many rooms
but the kitchen belongs to PawPaw

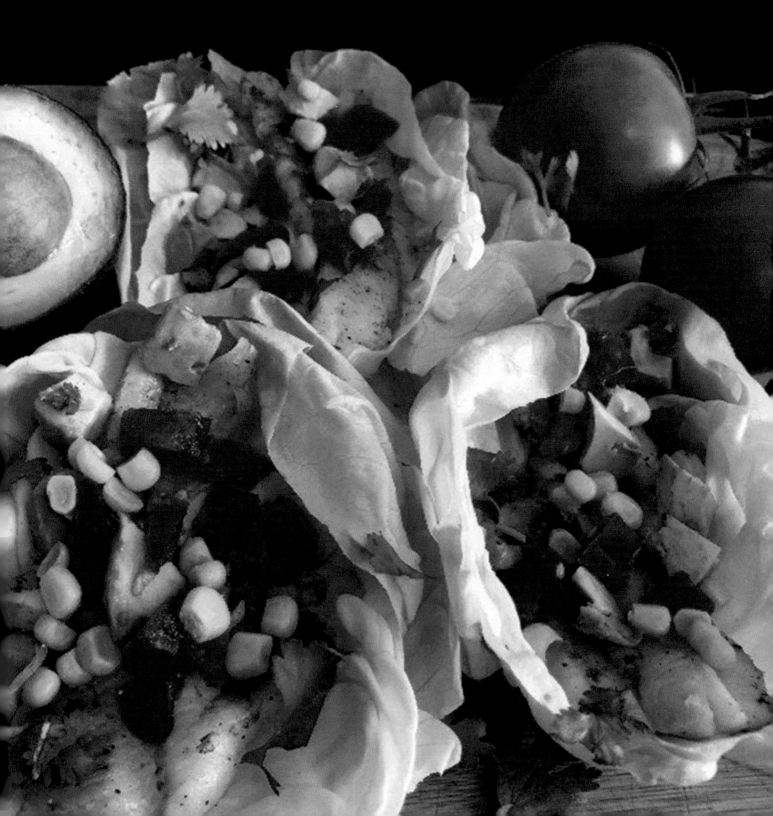

Cod Fish Lettuce Wrap

Cook time: 10 minutes

Servings: 2

Ingredients:

- 12 oz white fish
- 2 cups tomatoes, diced
- ¼ cup fresh cilantro, chopped
- 1 tablespoon olive oil
- Salt, pepper, to taste

- 8 romaine lettuce leaves
- 2 tablespoons Parmesan, shredded
- 1/4 cup of corn.
- 1 cup diced avocado

Instructions:

1. Preheat oil in a skillet over medium heat. Season fish with salt and pepper.
2. Add fish to the skillet and cook for 2-3 minutes per side. Chop the cooked fish.
3. Top each lettuce leave with fish, tomatoes, corn, avocado, cilantro and cheese.

Nutritional info (per serving): 220 calories; 10 g fat; 13 g total carbs; 18 g protein

Tequila Lime Fish Tacos

Cooking time: 30 minutes

Servings: 3

Ingredients:

To marinate the fish:

- 2 big fillets of tilapia (or 3 smaller ones)
- splash of olive oil
- splash of tequila
- a drizzle of agave syrup
- 1 clove garlic, chopped
- zest of 1 lime (you'll use the juice later)
- a few pinches of chile powder
- Salt, pepper, to taste

For the pickled onions:

- 1/2 red onion, thinly sliced
- splash of rice vinegar
- A few pinches of salt

To serve with:

- 6 corn or flour tortillas, grilled
- creme fraiche, sour cream, kewpie mayo.
- avocado slices
- sriracha
- shredded cabbage, seasoned with a little salt & lime juice
- cilantro
- extra lime slices

Instructions:

1. Whisk fish marinade ingredients together in a medium bowl. Coat fish and refrigerate for 30 minutes.

2. Thinly slice red onion.

3. Blanch slices in boiling water for 30 seconds and chill them immediately in ice water.

4. Drain and toss them with rice vinegar and salt.

5. Refrigerate until ready to use.

6. Heat the oven to 360F. Remove fish from the fridge. Cook it in the oven for 15-20 minutes. Squeeze a few big squeezes of lime juice on it just before you take it out of the oven. Let fish cool slightly, and flake it into smaller pieces.

7. Grill tortillas (or char them slightly over a gas flame).

8. Assemble tacos with the fish, a dollop of cream (of your choice), avocado slices, sriracha, shredded cabbage, cilantro, and serve with extra lime slices.

Nutritional info (per serving): 228 calories; 8.5 g fat; 25.5 g carbohydrate; 16.2 g protein

I like to consider myself a full meal with three sides

Sip like a Trophy Model

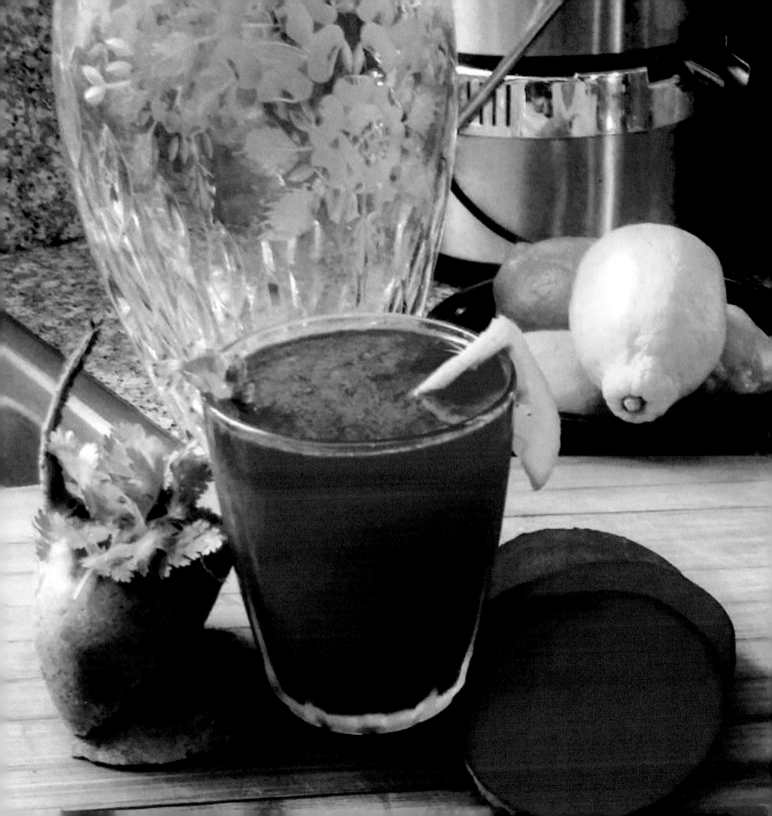

$\mathcal{B}$eets Slimming Juice

Cooking time: 5 minutes

Servings: 2

Ingredients:

- 1 beet, chopped
- 2 red cabbage leaves
- 3 medium carrots, chopped
- ½ lemon, sliced

- 1 orange, cut into wedges
- ¼ pineapple, chopped
- A handful spinach

Instructions:

1. Add all the ingredients to a blender or a food processor and process until smooth.
2. Pour into chilled glasses and serve.

Nutritional info (per serving): 121 calories; 0.3 g fat; 29.7 g carbohydrate; 2.9 g protein

Raspberry Cheesecake Smoothie

Cooking time: 5 minutes

Servings: 2

Ingredients:

- 2 cups frozen raspberries
- 1 cup unsweetened almond milk
- 1 ½ cup low fat cottage cheese

- 1 avocado, chopped
- 2 ripe frozen bananas, peeled, chopped
- 1 teaspoon vanilla extract

Instructions:

1. Add all the ingredients to a blender. Process until smooth.
2. Add the glasses to a freezer and chill before serving. Pour the smoothie into the glasses and serve.

Nutritional info (per serving): 407 calories; 16 g fat; 49 g carbohydrate; 23 g protein

Green Lemonade Blitz

Cooking time: 5 minutes

Servings: 2

Ingredients:

- 2 cups spinach
- 1 lemon
- 4 kale leaves
- 1 cucumber, diced
- 2 apples, diced

Instructions:

1. Add all the ingredients to your juicer.

2. Process the mixture until smooth and serve on top of ice.

Nutritional info (per serving): 175 calories; 0.8 g fat; 44.5 g carbohydrate; 4 g protein

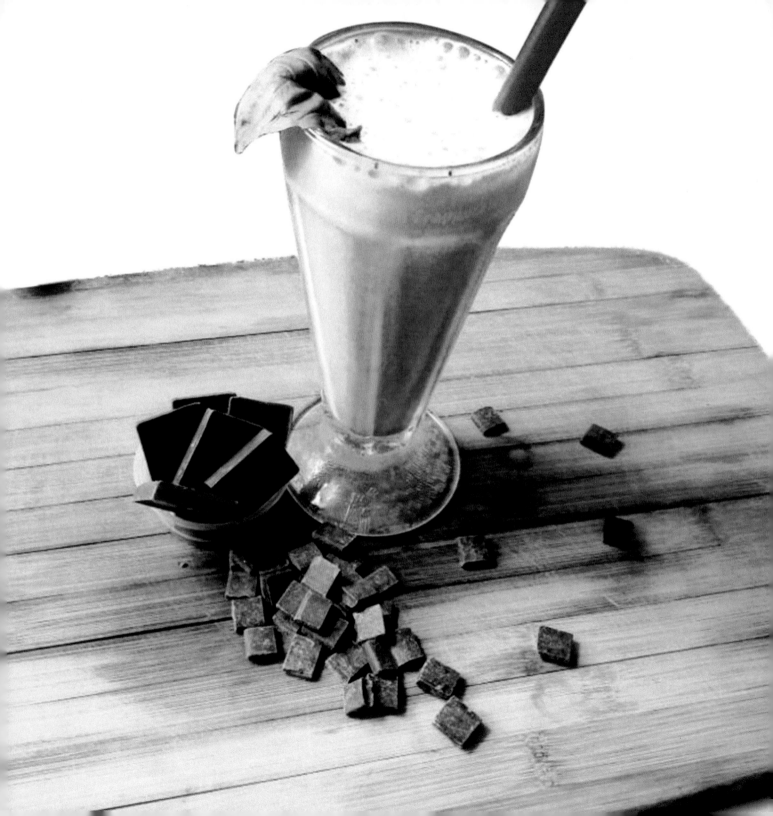

Protein Shake

Cook time: 5 minutes

Servings: 2

Ingredients:

- ¾ cup almond milk
- 2 tablespoons almond butter
- ½ cup ice
- 2 tablespoons unsweetened cocoa powder
- 2 tablespoons sweetener

- 1 tablespoon chia seeds
- 2 tablespoons hemp seeds
- ½ tablespoon pure vanilla extract
- A pinch of salt

Instructions:

1. Add all the ingredients to a blender and process until smooth.
2. Pour the shake into chilled glasses and serve topped with more chia and hemp seeds.

Nutritional info (per serving): 215 calories; 16.6 g fat; 25.9 g carbohydrate; 19.7 g protein

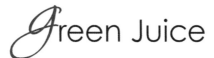reen Juice

Cook time: 5 minutes

Servings: 2

Ingredients:

- 3 apples, diced
- 3 celery stalks, diced
- ½ cucumber, diced
- ½ piece ginger, chopped
- 4 kale leaves
- 1 lemon
- 1 orange, peeled

Instructions:

1. Add all the ingredients to a blender and process until smooth.
2. Pour into chilled glasses and serve.

Nutritional info (per serving): 259 calories; 1 g fat; 27 g carbohydrate; 3.8 g protein

$\mathcal{B}$eet Cleansing Juice

Cook time: 5 minutes

Servings: 2

Ingredients:

- 3 celery stalks, chopped
- ½ inch ginger piece, chopped
- ½ cucumber, chopped
- 4 carrots, diced
- 1 beet, diced
- 2 apples, diced

Instructions:

1. Add all the ingredients to a blender and process until smooth.
2. Pour into chilled glasses and serve.

Nutritional info (per serving): 205 calories; 0.6 g fat; 21.6 g carbohydrate; 3.1 g protein

Red Spicy Blend

Cook time: 5 minutes

Servings: 2

Ingredients:

- 2 cups spinach
- ½ lime
- 1 jalapeno, chopped

- 2 celery stalks, chopped
- 5 carrots, chopped
- 1 beetroot, peeled, chopped

Instructions:

1. Add all the ingredients to a blender or a juicer and process until smooth.
2. Pour into chilled glasses and serve.

Nutritional info (per serving): 101 calories; 0.3 g fat; 23.8 g carbohydrate; 3.3 g protein

Superfood is the way to my heart

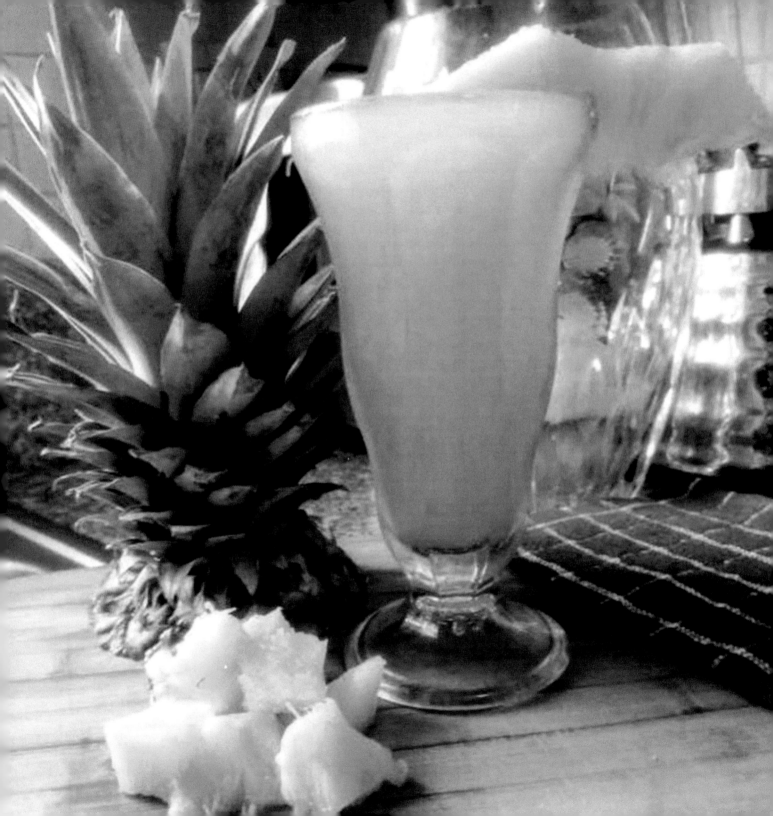

Pineapple Sunrise

Cook time: 5 minutes

Servings: 2

Ingredients:

- ¼ pineapple, peeled, chopped
- 4 kale leaves
- 2 celery stalks, chopped
- 4 large lettuce leaves
- 1 handful parsley

- 1 handful curly parsley
- 1 lemon, peeled and chopped
- 1 inch piece ginger
- 1 inch piece turmeric
- 1 chili pepper

Instructions:

1. Add all the ingredients to a blender or a juicer and process until smooth.
2. Pour into chilled glasses and serve.

Nutritional info (per serving): 51 calories; 0.4 g fat; 12.1 g carbohydrate; 2 g protein

Broccoli Weigh Loss Juice

Cook time: 5 minutes

Servings: 2

Ingredients:

- 1 broccoli stem, chopped
- 1 handful cilantro
- ½ cucumber, peeled, seeded and chopped
- 1 cup dark leafy greens
- 1 tablespoon lemon juice
- ½ cup water

Instructions:

1. Add all the ingredients to a blender or a juicer and process until smooth.
2. Pour into chilled glasses and serve.

Nutritional info (per serving): 49 calories; 0.3 g fat; 9.4 g carbohydrate; 3.3 g protein

So whether you eat or drink, whatever you do, do it for the glory of God-1 Corinthians 10:31 (NIV)

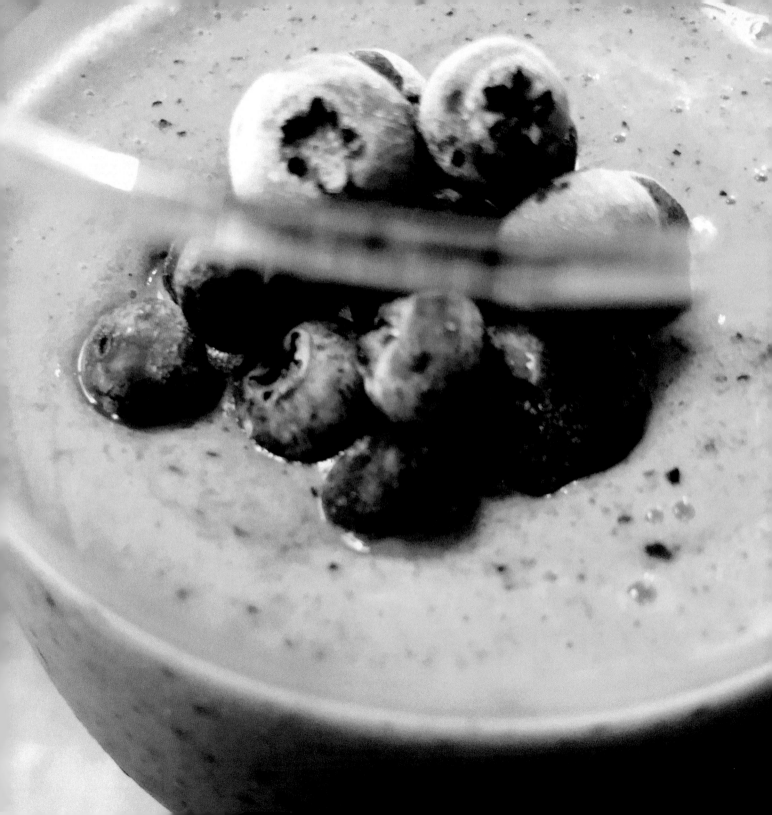

Blueberry Blitz

[[insert image 31]]

Cook time: 5 minutes

Servings: 2

Ingredients:

- 1 cup blueberries
- 8 oz yogurt
- 2 tablespoons sugar
- ¾ cup milk, reduced fat
- ½ teaspoon vanilla extract
- A pinch of nutmeg

Instructions:

1. Add all the ingredients to a blender or a juicer and process until smooth.
2. Pour into chilled glasses and serve.

Nutritional info (per serving): 211 calories; 3.9 g fat; 35.5 g carbohydrate; 9.5 g protein

$\mathcal{L}$ook Like a Trophy Model

Your Metabolism

It is quite easy to understand what metabolism is since everyone talks about it all the time. Metabolism is a process of converting food calories into energy needed for our bodies. Metabolism begins with digestion then goes into physical activity, and ends with a person breathing in sleep, when the body autonomously supplies oxygen to various organs.

What affects metabolism:

- body composition (the more the muscle mass, the faster the metabolism)
- gender (men have 5-10% faster metabolism)
- age (metabolism slows down with age)
- food thermogenesis (energy that body need to digest food)
- physical activity (the total number of calories you spend daily doing any activity).

How to make metabolism faster:

1. Drink more water

Water helps make metabolism faster by up to 3%. The daily consumption norm of water should be 0.61 fluid ounce per 1 pound of the body mass.

2. Eat often in small portions

You need to eat 4-6 times a day every 3 hours. People that have regular snacks generally eat less. And do not go hungry, as hunger slows down metabolic processes.

3. Add protein to your diet.

Lean protein helps make metabolism faster, because when digested, body spends twice as many calories to process it.

4. Eat food that makes metabolism faster

Eat food that makes metabolism faster. Citrus fruits, ginger, cinnamon, red hot pepper, green tea and coffee (no more than 3 cups a day), whole grain cereals, broccoli to name a few. Also eat food containing omega-3 fatty acids: fish fatty varieties like mackerel, herring, salmon, linseed oil, rice oil, nuts.

5. Breakfast

Anyone who refuses breakfast will never speed up his/her metabolism and will not lose weight. It is breakfast that gives a kick to metabolism.

6. Healthy sleep

In order to accelerate metabolism, you need to sleep at least 8 hours a day. Remember, if you do not sleep for a sufficient amount of time, it will be impossible to make the metabolism faster.

Intermittent Fasting

Intermittent fasting is a diet and an eating pattern that allows eating only at a certain time. It doesn't specify the exact food you should avoid, but rather tells when you should eat. Common intermittent fasting method that is used involves 16-hour fasts every day or fasting for the 24 hours once or twice per week. For the rest of the time that you are not allowed to eat you should forget about food, having limited yourself to drinking only water or vegetable and fruit juices in soft versions of the diet.

Fasting has been practiced throughout the human history. Pre historic hunter-gatherers didn't have food available all the time and sometimes they would stay without food for some time. As a result, humans evolved and learned to live without food or with small amount of food for extended periods of time. Knowing that fasting from time to time seems to be more natural than eating 3–4 (or more) meals a day.

Scientist investigated the process of autophagy, the mechanism of living cells getting rid of defective proteins and organelles. In the process of observation, scientists found out that the degree of autophagy, the rate of disposal of accumulated "debris", depends on the energy level in the cells. When energy is low, it destroys damaged or old proteins more intensively, making them a source of energy.

There are several most popular methods of intermittent fasting:

The 16/8 method, also called the Leangains protocol, involves skipping breakfast and limiting your daily eating time to 8 hours, which means you can eat for 8 hours and then you need to fast for 16 hours in between.

Eat-Stop-Eat which involves fasting for 24 hours, once or twice a week, which means not eating for whole 24 hours.

The 5:2 diet, which allows you to consume only 500–600 calories on two non-consecutive days of the week, but eat normally the other 5 days.

Low Carb Eating

A low-carb diet is an eating regimen that restricts the amounts of carbs, for example, sugars, pasta, and bread. It has a ton of protein, fat and sound vegetables. Now a lot of different low carb diets exist, and studies show that low carb diets can lead to weight reduction and improve in the overall wellbeing.

When choosing a low carb that is right for you and what foods to consume, you should think about your health, how much and how regularly do you exercise and how much weight you need to lose.

You can eat fish, eggs, vegetables, fruits, nuts, seeds, high-fat dairy foods, fats, healthy oils. Try not to eat: sugar, HFCS, wheat, vegetable oils, trans fats, "dietary" and low-fat foods and foods with a high level of processing.

You need to avoid the following foods and nutrients:

- Foods with a high level of processing: in case they seem to be made in an industrial facility, better avoid them.
- Refined grains: wheat, rice, barley and rye, just as bread, oats and pasta.
- Diet and low-fat foods: big number of dairy foods, cereals or crackers are low in fat, but have added sugar in them.
- Sugar: soda drinks, juices, agave, candy, ice cream and numerous different foods containing sugar.
- Starchy vegetables. It would be smarter to restrict the consumption of starchy vegetables if you are trying to reduce the intake of carbohydrates.
- Trans fats: hydrogenated or somewhat hydrogenated oils.

If you want to really follow a low-carb diet you should consider eating these organic, unprocessed low-carb foods:

- Vegetables: spinach, broccoli, cauliflower, carrots and many others.
- Nuts and seeds: almonds, walnuts, sunflower seeds, etc.
- Fats and oils: coconut oil, butter, olive oil and fish oil.
- Fruits: apples, oranges, pears, blueberries, strawberries.
- Fish: salmon, trout, haddock and many others; best trapped fish.
- High-fat dairy products: cheese, butter, heavy cream, yogurt.
- Eggs: Omega-3 fortified or grazing organic eggs are the best.

Try to eat as much organic products as you can every day.

$\mathcal{F}$it like a Trophy Model

Home Workout

You are thinking about getting fit, but you cannot find a suitable gym, the health club can be too expensive, or you already have a gym membership, but your schedule is just too hard. And you are not alone. Many people are now enjoying training at home in their own home gyms.

But can you really get the same or even better results as you would in a gym without leaving your home? Leading fitness experts say that it is absolutely possible to achieve great results by exercising at home. They even say they encourage people to be training at home, as it does not take much effort or resources to be training effectively at home. All you need is a fit ball, some dumbbells, exercise bands and push-up bars and a perfect gym is set. But the most important thing to have is consistency, which means you have to train regularly to make it a habit or even a lifestyle.

People prefer to train at home due to a large number of reasons. But regardless of those reasons you will need to make some preparations in order to make your home workouts most efficient you can get. So here are some tips to make you train better:

Make sure to plan everything ahead by making a to-do list by selecting the exact exercises you would like to do.

You need to be walking at least 8,000 steps or 3.5 miles a day. This number is perfect for your body and is easy on your limbs and joints.

You need to stay properly hydrated. You need to drink at least 1/3 of your body weight in ounces of water per day.

Create a designated fitness space so it is easier for you to train there and get into the mood.

Have a few go-to workouts memorized or ready all the time. You can do that by either downloading a phone app with some workout designed, stream workouts online and even get some DVDs.

One of the best workouts for fat loss and staying slim are also cardio and weight training. You can choose very simple cardio exercises and do them at home. Cardio exercises and weight training can even stop aging! Yes, it is not a myth. These exercises make your heart beat faster and they help your muscles to stay fit and toned longer. The recent studies showed that people who made cardio exercises regularly had significant improvements in their heart's performance.

The easiest cardio exercises you can do at home are:

- Running up and down the stairs
- Mountain climber exercise
- Jump squats
- Bicycle crunches
- Jumping with the rope

You can use Kettlebells or Resistance bands for the home weight training. They don't take a lot of space at home and you can use them any time, even 5-10 minutes of exercising will work for you! You don't even need equipment for this, just do squats or pushups and these easy exercises will help you stay fit and look young.

Thank you for choosing my book! I wish you good luck on your exciting journey to better health and lifestyle.

If you want to know more about Trophy Model's world, feel free to read my other book "Testimony of a Trophy Model: The Ugly Truth Behind the Beauty".

If you have any questions or comments do not hesitate to contact me

IG-@thetrophymodel

Email-thetrophymodel@gmail.com

IG-@EatlikeatrophymodelCover

Artwork by Sam McCain,

IG-steadyhandsammccain

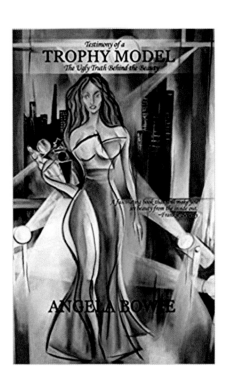

Yours

Angela Bowie

Printed in the United States
By Bookmasters